The Art of Tai Chi

Paul Crompton has studied Tai Chi and other martial arts for over twenty-five years and has been a teacher of Tai Chi for more than twenty years. He founded the *Karate and Oriental Arts* magazine in 1966 and has published seventy books on the different martial arts as well as producing videos on Tai Chi, Karate and Kung Fu.

The Art of Tai Chi

PAUL CROMPTON

ELEMENT

Shaftesbury, Dorset ● Rockport, Massachusetts
Brisbane, Queensland

© Paul Crompton 1993

Published in Great Britain in 1993 by
Element Books Limited
Longmead, Shaftesbury, Dorset

Published in the USA in 1993 by
Element, Inc.
42 Broadway, Rockport, MA 01966

Published in Australia in 1993 by
Element Books Limited for
Jacaranda Wiley Limited
33 Park Road, Milton, Brisbane, 4064

Cover design by Max Fairbrother
Design by Roger Lightfoot
Illustrations by Michael Cole
Typeset by Footnote Graphics, Warminster, Wiltshire
Printed and bound in Great Britain by
Redwood Books, Trowbridge, Wiltshire

British Library Cataloguing in Publication
data available

Library of Congress Cataloging in Publication
data available

ISBN 1–85230–430–8

20028360

Contents

Introduction: What is Tai Chi Chuan?   vii

1. Tai Chi and Philosophy   1
2. The Theory of Chi Kung   13
3. Aspects of Physics in Tai Chi   21
4. Principles of Tai Chi Chuan   27
5. Introductory Exercises   31
6. Learning the 48 Form Set of Tai Chi   40
7. Push Hands (Tui Shou)   85
8. Tai Chi Today   91

Further Reading   97
Useful Addresses   98
General Index   99
Index of Forms   100

Introduction: What is Tai Chi Chuan?

Everyone has seen movement in slow motion. When you see a film showing action slowed down, several things happen. One is that you can see more clearly what is taking place, and another is that sometimes the film sequence appears more dramatic. Tai Chi Chuan, usually abbreviated to Tai Chi or Taiji, is movement in slow motion. When you do Tai Chi, *you* slow down, *you* can see more clearly how you are moving, and you feel that *you* are in the picture. You are not being swept along by the rapids of ordinary, daily life, but entering a different time scale, and calmer, more placid waters. Life itself seems to slow down, and you have an opportunity to experience your own body in motion: relaxed, evenly spaced, more rooted to the ground, natural, unhurried.

Sounds good? Then read on, and be led into this different world, created and sustained by centuries of dedication by the people of China. China always was and still largely is an agricultural society. Most of the population worked the land, prayed for rain, witnessed the coming and going of the seasons, and were in general close to nature, as the saying goes. Many of their ideas, philosophical outlooks, patterns of behaviour, much of their cultural heritage in fact, are derived from observations and experiences of the natural world.

As more and more of the people in our times have moved into the cities, grown up and been educated in the cities, this contact with the natural world has become very weak and sporadic. We do call for 'green' reforms, for a reduction in pollution and so forth, but the basis for our concerns is information fed to us by the media. We do not live in the countryside; we do not experience it directly. So if a rurally based society offers us something which has a 'natural' origin, we should grasp it with both hands, and feet, as it contains more than a whiff of clean air and a very stabilizing tempo.

You may have seen film clips of people in the Far East moving very slowly and gracefully in parks and open spaces. The chances are that they were doing Tai Chi. They were performing sequences of movement, arranged in a definite order, at a uniform speed. Is that all, you may say? Well, yes, that is all; but there is much more to this 'all' than meets the uninformed eye. Every movement conforms to definite principles, sustained throughout the sequence. When practised with correctness and sufficient regularity, these principles can be absorbed, to some extent, by the student. The benefits of this can be considerable.

To get a better idea of this claim, consider your usual movements in life and the movements of friends and people you see at work and in the street. Generally everyone is rushing, pushing, reacting, under pressure, under stress. Even when we 'enjoy' ourselves it is often with a kind of frenzy. There is rarely a warm feeling of relaxation and an impression of having plenty of time to spare. The natural, rural world has a tempo of its own in which nothing can be rushed. The seeds in the earth must wait for the sun and the rain; the fruit of the trees must wait for the summer in order to ripen; the animals who hibernate must wait for the spring warmth, and so on. Early Chinese observers of life and early Chinese philosophers noted these obvious facts and tried to absorb them into their own lives, to some extent. Tai Chi can be seen as an expression of this attempt; an attempt which was successful. Its success can be seen in the way the movements of the art ebb and flow, like the waves, like the tides. The practitioner advances and retreats, turns left, turns right, rises and falls, and all this at a slow, measured speed which refuses to be hurried.

Once the sequences of Tai Chi have been learned, then the whole body, mind and spirit feels more harmonized, returning as it does to something more natural in itself. The joints of the body function more correctly; the muscles stretch and contract with a feeling of ease; the breathing gradually slows down and the brain loses for a while its burden of concerns. When this happens, say the Chinese followers of Tai Chi, the nectar of saliva is stimulated, helping the processes of digestion. All the restorative forces of the person begin to be mobilized and for a time one's life flows in the direction of repair and regeneration. Less obvious, and some may say more nebulous results may also follow, but these are described in the next chapter.

History

Imagine, if you will, a mountainous region in China. Gnarled, wild-branched trees cling to the sides of precipitous rocks. Mists float with almost imperceptible motion above bottomless chasms; and above the mists, from the mountain peaks, on all sides the land seems to stretch into infinity. Stalking through such a region, his seven foot, roughly clad frame giving pause even to the fiercest wild beasts, comes the Taoist immortal Chang San-feng. His eyes, piercing and deep as the abysses at his feet, see the markings on the wings of a distant insect. His hands, hanging loosely at his sides, have at one and the same time the sensitivity of a watchmaker and the power of a blacksmith. At one with nature, his immense force makes the air around him vibrate with Chi, vital energy, as though an invisible bellows were at work.

One evening, Chang San-feng lies down to sleep, for even he must rest. In his slumber he begins to dream. A heavenly presence demonstrates to him the fundamental movements of Tai Chi Chuan, the Supreme, Ultimate Way of the Fist. Awakening, Chang remembers what he has been shown, and realizes that he must impart this precious gift to humanity. As he travels he passes through a village. He learns that as many as one hundred brigands are plaguing the luckless inhabitants with impossible demands for food and clothing, women and money. He waits. When the brigands come again, Chang resorts to his Tai Chi movements, mobilizes an art of gentleness into an art of devastation, and like one of the raging dragons which live on the peaks of Wu-tang, he scatters them like autumn leaves. They never return.

Did Chang San-feng ever live at all? Scholars doubt it, lovers of legend do not. Did he create Tai Chi from a dream? Some believe it, but later evidence says he did not. Legend says he was a friend of a Taoist advisor to Kublai Khan, in the thirteenth century AD; that he miraculously made flowers grow and trees blossom in double quick time; that he shunned society and even avoided an audience with the emperor, during the fifteenth century. True or not, the very existence of the legends tends to elevate Tai Chi and make it something to be striven for. The association with Taoism seems to have persisted also, and eventually Tai Chi, as we know it today and as it exists in a plurality of forms in China, contains movements derived from martial arts, Kung fu, Wushu, and movements stemming from Taoist meditation and traditional Chinese medical knowledge. In these respects at least it relates to the story of Chang San-feng.

Throughout recorded Chinese history there was an interest in the study and systematization of methods of combat and exercise; the two overlapping very frequently. The famous treatise, *The Art of War*, written centuries ago by Sun Tzu is ample testimony to this. This systematization included the strategy and tactics of armies and methods of single combat. Wherever we dip into Chinese history there is always an individual or two striving with might and main to perfect a technique of swordsmanship, spearmanship, grappling, punching, wrestling, exercising, feats of strength and endurance. If you can imagine it, some Chinese man or woman was almost certainly doing it. For instance, there is a Chinese art of fighting using a wooden bench; an unarmed combat method which imitates the fighting movements of a chicken; a series of training methods for hunting tigers with a trident-shaped fork; the list is very long – no one knows how long. Of course not everyone by any means was interested in such things, and when they were not training the armies, fighting off brigands and generally helping those too weak to help themselves, it appears that martial artists, as we call them today, were often despised by the rest of the populace.

One such researcher and martial artist was Wang Tsung-yueh of Shansi. He knew an art of exercise and combat which apparently until his day, sometime in the late eighteenth century, had not been recorded. Once he went into a village belonging to the Chen family, in Honan province. He had the temerity to pass a disapproving remark about some martial arts training he had witnessed in the village and was promptly challenged to back up his words. He did so to such effect that the village leaders asked him to stay and teach them his art. Wang did stay and so passed on his Tai Chi Chuan, the Supreme, Ultimate Way of the Fist, to the Chen family. In this story, and at this stage of its development, Tai Chi shows no evidence of being the meditation in movement which we mainly know it as today. Its strength lay in the fact that with its help Wang had defeated members of the Chen family in single combat. This lends strength to the argument that side by side with the martial development of Tai Chi ran another stream of exercise derived from or practised by some Taoists and Chi Kung exponents (see Chapter 2). Later, it is thought the streams merged in certain respects, through the efforts of men such as Sun Lu-t'ang, Chen Wei-ming and Cheng Man-ch'ing, to name but a very few. If this is not the case, then where did the Tai Chi we have today, a blend of methods, ideas, theories and stories, come from?

The Chen family continued to train and develop their new art. They were influenced by other martial arts and different movements were added to what they had received from Wang Tsung-yueh. A member of the Yang family, Yang Lu-chan, studied with the Chen and later developed his own style of Tai Chi. One man and woman after another became interested in the art until today there are several styles, each usually bearing the family name of the founder, for example:

Chen style
Yang style
Old Wu style
New Wu style
Sun style
Hao style

Why the original style was changed into so many others is an interesting question. This tendency still persists; decried by some, encouraged by others. One explanation lies in the background of the men and women concerned. For instance, in the Sun style, named after Sun Lu-t'ang, Master Sun had also studied Pakua and Hsing-I. When in later life he had studied Tai Chi and wished to practise an art which was as it were 'his own' he brought into the movement sequence some of his favourite movements and methods from the other two arts. It was so highly thought of by his peers that it was named after him: Sun style. Other reasons for changes

in the style originally learned can be found in physical build
and temperament. A very tall, heavy person will tend
gradually to change what he or she has learned to suit his or
her physique. Similarly, a thin, wiry, quick-moving person
will do the same. Such people will tend to emphasize the
movements which suit them, maybe repeat them several
times and reduce the number of times the movements which
do not suit them are performed. Someone else may be more
interested in slow, calming movements and will emphasize
them; or be more interested in fighting and so introduce
more fighting techniques into a Form, and perhaps change
the speed. These and other variations are possible and in-
deed found within the range of Tai Chi sequences.

More material on the development of Tai Chi can be found
in my book, *The Elements of Tai Chi*. However, to give some
insight into how styles of Tai Chi and Chinese martial arts in
general sometimes develop and change, the following
account which is not in that book is included here.

After the terrible traumas of the Second World War and
the Communist Revolution in China, efforts were made
to collect what remained of the Chinese martial arts and
produce a syllabus which could be taught in schools and
colleges. Famous teachers assembled together with the
heads of education in the field of athletics and a Wushu
training system emerged. The emphasis was on athletic ability in many cases, and some of the old, martial, combative
techniques were dropped. This has been seen as a retrograde
step by many traditionalists, but, judged on its own merits
and not compared with anything else, the Wushu syllabus is
acrobatic, beautiful to watch and exhilarating to perform.

Among the contributors to the syllabus was Li Tian-ji,
famous with the sword and an experienced martial artist. An
important contribution which Li made was to develop the
Form of Tai Chi known as the Combined Form, not to be
confused with the Combined Form found in the latest (1992)
Wushu Syllabus. The latter Form is in fact the 48 Form Set
described in this book. The Combined Form, which is a long
sequence, consists of movements taken from other styles of
Tai Chi such as Yang and Chen, with more than a suggestion
of movements from Pakua and Hsing-I, the two companion
martial arts to Tai Chi. Even though Li Tian-ji put so much
into the creation of the Combined Form, it was left to one

Bow Sim Mark to make it popular. And it was not in China that this popularity spread but in the United States, to which Bow Sim Mark had emigrated. Some fifteen years or so after she had first introduced the Combined Form to a wider audience, Bow Sim Mark wrote a book on it, for which Li Tian-ji thanked her. Li himself wrote that whenever he remembered that it had been left to Bow Sim Mark to do this work he felt 'greatly ashamed'. This Combined Form, which I have practised for some six or seven years myself, lives on in pupils trained by Bow Sim Mark and in the first students of the 1950s in China. It can vary in speed in different sections of the sequence, and has hard, hitting movements as well as grace and slowness. It is not a Form for absolute beginners.

This example shows that like any living art form, Tai Chi is dynamic in the sense that it continues to develop. Its movements express principles. They can be done for exercise, for martial arts study, and can be adapted for self-defence close-quarter techniques.

Aspects

Apart from the martial aspect of Tai Chi, which is the one with which Westerners are least familiar, there is the quiet, meditative, solo aspect. It is this one which most readily comes to mind when the art is mentioned in conversation. Chi Kung is the most likely source of this strand; it will be explained more thoroughly in Chapter 2 but briefly Chi Kung means the cultivation, through persistent application and hard efforts of concentration, of the intrinsic energy of the body, its vitality, its . . . – the word does not exist for us as we do not have the concept. Vitality is for me an acceptable word. Through certain exercises and through using the imagination and mental concentration, Chi Kung practitioners try to spread out more evenly through the body the vital energy necessary to keep the body healthy. They also try to store this energy in specific points or centres in the body. One could say that through exercise and concentration they try to do what acupuncturists do with their needles and moxa.

As in the case of the origin of Tai Chi itself, the origin of

Chi Kung is lost. Writings of at least two thousand years ago contain references to Chi Kung, and historians of the subject see a thread of the art running continuously through China since those early times. A well-known tradition speaks of Bodhidharma, an Indian monk who founded the Ch'an school of Buddhism in China, coming to that country in the sixth century AD. Monks under his direction were so weak that he devised a system of Chi Kung exercises known as the Yi Chin Ching to make them more fit and healthy, better able to withstand the rigours of the spiritual life. The system, it is claimed, exists today in the same form as it did some 1,400 years ago. The exercises are mainly stretching, combined with breathing and concentration. Another well-known system of Chi Kung is called the Eight Pieces of Brocade; the movements consist of stretching, loosening the joints, breathing and concentration. In modern times a popular system called Wild Goose Chi Kung has been written and talked about with some enthusiasm. Its movements are far stronger and more elaborate than either of the other two.

Tai Chi is itself sometimes referred to as an example of Chi Kung. This is an accurate description, in a sense, but its qualification for this description depends largely on the manner in which it is done. If the sequence is performed slowly, evenly, in a relaxed way, paying attention to detail and following the principles, then it can be described as Chi Kung. If it is done with stops and starts, emphasizing power in certain places and generally elaborating on the martial arts applications, then the name Chi Kung needs qualification. Chi Kung is sometimes divided into two: internal and external. The internal does not, as its name obviously suggests, put as much emphasis on the strength of the muscles of the body, on external effect and so on as does external Chi Kung.

My own attitude to the use of the expression Chi Kung, for what it's worth, is that it should be reserved for internal Chi Kung. The reason for this is that Chi Kung should be undertaken with a maximum use of intelligence and a minimum use of tension and brute force. We in the West have the equivalent of external Chi Kung, hard Chi Kung. But we have not had the equivalent of internal Chi Kung, at least not in any readily available sense. Scientific athletic training, even non-scientific or entirely subjective home-made athletic training, is a form of external Chi Kung. It uses mental concentration, muscle power, knowledge of anatomy and breathing to produce the energy to bring about the desired result. The aim, the end, is for an external result: winning, beating someone else, and so on. Internal Chi Kung is for the performer or practitioner alone, aiming for some kind of internal balance of Chi, leading to a different outlook, even to moments of enlightenment.

If you study Tai Chi you will come across different outlooks or similar outlooks to the ones mentioned above. With experience you will find your own views, methods and favourite movements.

1. Tai Chi and Philosophy

The book mentioned earlier, *The Elements of Tai Chi*, attempts to question the rational connections between certain philosophical ideas common in Chinese history and Tai Chi training and study. A great deal has been written about the connection between the two, and much of it does not bear up under critical examination. Some martial artists, influenced by Western methods of thought, have, in recent years, questioned and even condemned attempts to relate difficult, subtle and abstruse ideas with Tai Chi and Pakua training. They said that martial artists could be divided into two types; the doers, the body guards, the effective fighters and explorers into the practical development of the arts, and the scholar martial artists who did study in a practical way, but who felt compelled to try to connect perennial Chinese philosophies with martial arts in ways which stretched one's powers of belief, to say the least, and at times verged on the fantastic. Since some of these criticisms come from Chinese martial artists, this does show that a critical attitude towards trying to carry the relationship between Tai Chi and philosophy too far is not simply a product of Western rationalism, but has some sympathy among the Chinese themselves.

This chapter leaves all such debate aside and as straightforwardly as possible presents some of the philosophy which the majority of Tai Chi students find when they attend classes and read the literature. This will leave readers, in the light of experience, to examine what is said for themselves.

Over two thousand years ago there were so many systems of philosophy in China that they were known as 'the hundred schools'. Taoism and Buddhism were two among many and had no particular prominence. Gradually these two schools became very important, along with the teachings of Confucius and his philosophical descendants. Another school, the Yin-Yang, is sometimes merged with Taoism, but originally was a separate system.

Taoism

Taoism is linked with the man Lao Tzu, and the famous book popularly attributed to him, the *Tao Te Ching*. The title means the 'Classic of the Way and the Power'. The opening words of the book are: 'The Tao that can be expressed in words is not the eternal (real) Tao'. The Tao is that which 'causes' all things to come into existence. We do not understand what it is, and the name itself, Tao, is not its name. We give it a name merely to indicate that it is. Creation itself simply *is*, using Tao as an inexplicable cause: 'From Tao comes one; from one comes two; from two comes three and from three comes all things'.

A widespread idea in Chinese philosophy is that when any process reaches its extreme, it begins to return or reverse. For instance when water boils and reaches its maximum temperature it turns into steam, cooling, condensing, becoming once again cold or cooler water. When a fever in a sick person reaches a certain pitch, the body sweats, the fever 'breaks' and the person's temperature, it is to be hoped, returns to normal. Like so many statements in Chinese thought there are many everyday examples to support the basic idea behind them. The *Tao Te Ching* has a statement supporting the idea of the elastic nature of an extreme condition when it says that; 'Returning (or reversing) is the movement of the Tao'.

One of the attributes of a follower of the teachings of the *Tao Te Ching* is that he or she is alert to, aware of, compliant with the presence of extremes. This awareness governs their actions so that they recognize that if they do not 'contend, then no one can contend with them'. If they are not aggressive they will not reach the extreme of aggressiveness. In Tai Chi there is an exercise called Push Hands (See Chapter 7), done with a partner. In a prearranged fashion first one student pushes the other and in turn is pushed back. The initial idea of this exercise is that each student learns to yield, give way, that is, not 'contend'. When pushed he or she senses the pressure of the push and gives way, keeping contact; the person pushing senses this yielding and does not push too far, otherwise his or her 'going to extremes' will cause him or her to lose balance. So first the one and then the other student advances and retreats, not going too far. Of course there is some contention, but without it there would be no learning! A striking thing about the fundamental, early teachings of Taoism is that they contain statements almost identical to some of the statements made by Jesus Christ, and other figures in the New Testament.

> Except ye be converted, and become as little children, ye shall not enter into the kingdom of heaven.
>
> Gospel according to St Matthew

> Can you have the softness and resilience of a breathing child?
>
> Tao Te Ching

Another common expression in Taoism is 'Wu-wei' which can be translated as 'non-action, not having any activity', or even, 'doing nothing'. Some critics of Eastern philosophy have jumped on this expression and said that it leads people in the direction of an aimless, listless life-style. This is to misunderstand the idea behind the expression. Wu-wei follows from the practice of not going to extremes. Modern commentators have explained this by saying that it means that we should do something but must always be careful not to overdo it. Telling little Jimmy to try to keep his clothes clean is all right as a pointer. Nagging him repeatedly on every occasion will probably either make him react by finally rolling in mud or produce a little boy who is so busy keeping clean that he never enjoys himself throughout his childhood, with disastrous results perhaps when he becomes an adult!

The second word in *Tao Te Ching* is 'Te'. It means something such as power, virtue or intrinsic natural strength. A man or woman in touch with Tao experiences natural power or virtue; that which is natural to them, their Te. Te aligns a person with the world, with life, guided by the Tao. Such a person does not need to be given arbitrary rules and regulations; Te is his or her guide. Thus, a life guided by Te is simple; not naive or that of a simpleton, but uncomplicated by the unnecessary, by extremes.

This attitude contrasted very much with the humanist qualities taught by Confucius. In his book, Lao Tzu rated humanist virtues lower down the scale:

> Tao should guide us
> but if the Tao is lost
> we have Te;
> if Te is lost
> we have humanist virtues;
> if humanist virtues are lost
> we have a feeling for what is righteous;
> if a feeling for what is righteous is lost
> we have ceremonial;
> and ceremonial is the beginning of chaos.

The development of this theme brings in ideas which are very much out of keeping with our times, when the notion of education for everyone to the highest possible academic and technical level is the order of the day. When we educate people we fill their minds with knowledge, ideas, theories, aims and desires which they cannot possibly fulfil; contact with Te is lost, and the received content of education replaces it. To obtain their desires people become more cunning, less truthful, less reliable, more devious, and so not only is contact with Te lost but contact with humanistic virtues and then with righteous feelings. Such people have to be governed by iron laws, which they try to break or circumvent, and society crumbles. The people perish because they have lost contact with their root.

In Tai Chi the notion of a root is first of all approached in a purely physical sense. Students first learn to keep their balance, by standing and stepping in certain ways which keep the lower abdomen where the centre of gravity should be. They are encouraged to let their awareness go down, out of their head and thoughts and into the abdomen and legs. They begin to feel more rooted, better based, more centred. If they persist in training they may begin to see the connection between tension and the loss of rootedness: this brings into focus various anxieties and fears which cause the tensions. They begin to see that going to extremes in physical movements is the manifestation of an attitude, an emotional condition. They may then begin to reflect in a more holistic way about life in general. They may; there again they may not . . .

Lao Tzu makes reference to the innocence and naturalness of children before they are contaminated by grown-ups. He praises this child-like condition and asks us if we too can become like little children. This is one of the sayings that remind one of the sayings of Jesus Christ when he said that unless we become like little children we shall not enter the Kingdom of Heaven. We could hazard a guess that both Christ and Lao Tzu may have been referring to the same thing; that contact with Te was like being a little child, and that the Kingdom of Heaven was like contact with the Tao. A Chinese saying is that 'Great wisdom is like ignorance'. Innocence is a form of ignorance, yet it does not mean stupidity or a lack in knowledge. It means knowing what is necessary, and not being cluttered up with what is not necessary.

Chuang Tzu

Chuang Tzu is another famous early Taoist who came after Lao Tzu. One of his works is called *The Happy Journey or Excursion*. In it he speaks about what is natural and what is not. By natural he means what is innate, and by what is not natural he means what is not innate. He cites the example of a horse, which by nature has four legs; what is not natural to a horse is for it to have a saddle and bridle. If we try to shorten the legs of a crane we cannot do it, except by cutting them off; and if we try to lengthen the legs of a duck we shall only do so by painfully stretching them. When we change what is natural, therefore, we should always exercise caution.

In Tai Chi training a student tries to see what is natural in his or her movements. Though the movements of Tai Chi are in a sense not natural, that is, they have been introduced from the outside, this is justifiable because the usual movements of civilized people are even further from what is natural. Therefore, Tai Chi movements help to restore what is natural. In the end, as it were, one can dispense with Tai Chi movements, having found once again what one had as a child. In fact, few if any students achieve this; it is more common that they simply give up!

Chuang Tzu's teachings point directly, as did Lao Tzu's before him, to a growing intimacy with the workings of nature and of the universe itself. Even this happy journey is a relative one; and this should be borne in mind. He tells the story of a man called Lieh Tzu whose efforts to understand himself and whose pursuit of the natural had brought him to a state in which he could ride on the wind. But of course he had not reached a state of independence for he was subject to the existence and whims of the wind. When the wind blew he could travel, and then only; or, he had to walk! Beyond this state of dependence is another, in which a person is, as it is said, at one with the universe, and feels no distinction which cuts him or her off from the universe.

Tai Chi may point its followers towards something like this, as a goal, but it begins by trying to be at one with one's own body, in motion. To do this one must see what is unnatural, what is unnecessary and begin to ride on the wind of one's own momentum, one's own weight and body structure; not stuck in the mud of one's own tensions and ego, one's contentiousness. Following this direction a person can begin to question not only their movements but also their opinions. In expressing their opinions a person contends with other opinions and if their opinions prevail they say that they are right and the other person is wrong. They feel more and more that they are right, that they are always right and others are wrong, except for the ones who agree with them, who, of course, are right also. Their attitude becomes extreme, like the attitudes of politicians, and they are in danger.

The Taoist view as described by Chuang Tzu transcends the personal opinion because it sees that there are many points of view, many angles to any question. It also sees that what a person may believe strongly today they may disavow tomorrow. Taoism sees change, another strong idea in Chinese philosophy, whereas ordinary people see or believe in fixed opinions, fixed situations, fixed relationships. By seeing life from this position, the Taoist adept has no position, no opinion which they cling to, and so has no territory to defend, nothing to contend about. Every occasion is unique.

In doing Push Hands with such a philosophical attitude, Tai Chi students can perceive that at one second they are pushing and at another they are yielding. The constant movement of the exercise indicates to them that there is no fixed place which they can use for defence. They are in constant motion, a piece in an ever-changing pattern. So they have nothing to defend, nothing to lose and also nothing to gain. These ideas are so alien to most Western civilization and upbringing that it is difficult for them to find even the smallest foothold even in Tai Chi training, let alone our lives. However, the finger is there, pointing, and we can remember that at least. In case the Taoist teaching, such as presented above, seems empty and nihilist to readers, here is another explanation of the Taoist path. When they begin, would-be adepts look at the world and see people, trees, cities, and all the things of life; then as they go on they become completely uncertain about what they see, what they know, what they do. They are filled with a kind of doubt. At last, they pass through this to a state of enlightenment, in which they have forgotten their doubt and forgotten their original certainty. They are no longer the person who was so certain about everything, nor the person who was uncertain. They are someone else. What that is, only they know.

Yin and Yang

Though in later centuries the idea of Yin and Yang, the Opposites, seemed to merge with later forms of Taoism, and in most writings in English are spoken of in the same breath, the Yin-Yang School was originally distinct from Taoism. Translation into English of Chinese terms is often very difficult to do accurately, because the cultures and outlooks are so different. It has been said for instance that the Yin-Yang School originated from Chinese occultists. But to Western minds, what does this mean? Perhaps the word 'occultists' conjures up a wide range of meanings from people who use ouija boards, read tea leaves, believe mumbo-jumbo, seriously and sincerely try to understand the Kabbalah, and so on. Occultists is such a loaded word. If we take it to its root, we find that it concerns things which are hidden. Whatever the meaning of occultists, the early Chinese variety were interested in astrology, in finding an accurate calendar, in the 'five elements', in divination such as is found in the

I-Ching, in physiognomy, in geomancy, and in similar subjects.

Of these subjects, the one which has had the greatest influence on Tai Chi theory is the notion of the five elements. One of the key areas of Chinese scholarship in which the number five is found is in the study of history. At the appearance of the universe everything divided into five elements or five powers. The different dynasties of China were grouped in accordance with the prevalence of one of the powers. At the time of the legendary Yellow Emperor the element earth was in the ascendant; during the Hsia dynasty the element wood; in the Shang dynasty the element metal; in the Chou dynasty the element fire, and, in writings attributed to T'sou Yen, the next dynasty would be governed by the element water. To like-minded Chinese philosopher-historians it was in the order of things that dynasties would rise and fall, since one of the five elements is always succeeded by another, dominating the other. As each element waxes it must wane and fall under the influence of the next. An element can also be seen as something which gives rise to its successor. Water gives rise to wood; wood gives rise to fire; fire gives rise to earth; earth gives rise to metal and metal gives rise to water. The cycle continues. Each element has its corresponding colour. Chinese emperors who believed in the five element theory would take on the colour of their element as the royal colour. The Yellow Emperor had yellow as his colour, corresponding to earth; the Chou Emperor lived in a period of water domination so took black as his colour.

Some Tai Chi students and teachers made connections between the five elements and the performance of the forms. Advancing corresponded to metal, retreating to wood, looking left to water, looking right to fire, and being in equilibrium to earth. By analysing each movement they found it possible to relate it to the elements. In Push Hands and in the application of Tai Chi to combat, it was possible to show that different techniques would overcome the actions of other techniques not simply in reality but also according to the succession of the five elements. So a technique corresponding to water would overcome a technique which corresponded to fire. This process of structuring Tai Chi according to the five elements is a complicated affair, and its detail is not appropriate to an introductory book such as this.

The five element theory provided philosophers and historians with an explanation of the universe's structure, but did not explain how the universe was created in the first place. The Yin-Yang School itself did that. Originally the word Yang stood for sunshine, and then the light side of a hill or mountain. The word Yin meant darkness, where the sun was not shining, or shadow. Gradually this purely descriptive use of the two words changed into an abstract one also, and Yang became an active principle, Yin a passive principle. These two principles, manifesting as opposite forces, created the universe. Later still, the two words were used in connection with a process of divination provided by the *I-Ching, Book of Changes*. An unbroken or strong line —— signified the Yang influence and two broken lines – – the Yin influence. In any situation the relative predominance and grouping of the lines indicated something about the outcome of any question which the diviner was asking.

The picture shows the fundamental trigrams of the I-Ching. These were later changed into tiers of six lines giving sixty-four hexagrams. Tai Chi theorists attributed the tiers to physical techniques of their art, along with their corresponding five element designation. Readers will appreciate that this became a complicated process.

During the eleventh century AD, Chou Tun-yi, a Taoist, studied some of the diagrams used by religious Taoists, as distinct from philosophers, to show in pictorial form how immortality could be achieved. From his studies, Chou produced the diagram which is now equated with Tai Chi. This is called the Supreme Ultimate. Its white side shows the Yang principle and its black side the Yin principle. The small dot of the opposite colour signifies that nothing is completely Yang or Yin; there is always a trace of Yin in Yang, and Yang in Yin. The symbol also shows that as one force diminishes the other grows. The symbol is used by Tai Chi students to show how aggressive force is diminished by yielding, and how yielding too has its limits – in any direction – and unless changed will fall to aggressive force. For instance, if someone pushes you, and you yield, if you do so in a straight line and the aggressive force is increased or continues, you must circle. That is, you must turn away to one side, or lose balance.

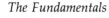

The Fundamentals

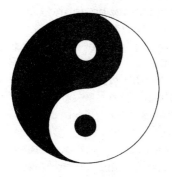

The Supreme Ultimate

The whole performance of a Tai Chi sequence can be interpreted as an interplay of Yin and Yang; the positions of the palms, upward facing or downward facing, can be so interpreted, as can the fullness, weight bearing, or emptiness, non-weight bearing, of the feet. Breathing in and breathing out can be seen in the same way. For those who like this kind of intellectual explanation the Yin-Yang theory is fascinating. It gives one some insight into the idea of change, the root idea of the I-Ching, and reinforces the Taoist ideal of submitting to change and having as one's goal to be at one with the universe.

Ch'an Buddhism

Tradition has it that some time in the sixth century AD a Buddhist monk, Bodhidharma, made the perilous journey to China and transmitted an esoteric teaching to Hui-k'o. What he transmitted was an approach to enlightenment from the Buddha himself who, when asked a serious question by one of his followers, held up a flower and smiled. This particular teaching was passed on at that moment, through the flower, the smile, the Buddha. Since that time it has remained separate from the so-to-speak 'theology' of Buddhism, the sermons, the long treatises, the discussions, the definitions. From India it passed to China and from China to Japan, where it is known as Zen Buddhism.

The teaching of Bodhidharma fell on the fertile ground created by the Taoists, who already had something similar. The *Tao Te Ching*, if nothing else, indicates this. The meeting of the two produced Ch'an. Defining Ch'an is a contradiction in terms. It is something which cannot be defined. As has been said in this respect, when you try to catch it, it is no longer there. Interestingly enough, much has been said and written about this indefinable something. This is partly because the Ch'an teacher recognizes the difficulties for his or her pupils in studying anything without the use of words. He or she tries to lead the pupils, perhaps through words, to a point where they see the uselessness of words and for only an instant, perhaps, the words fall away and the pupil perceives something real and true, directly. He or she experiences, instead of thinks. Inevitably, when the experience is over, words come back and the process begins again. Thus, although the preparation for enlightenment may be long and arduous, the experience itself is described as sudden. The Ch'an School has been called the School of Sudden Enlightenment.

Bodhidharma is considered by many of the followers of Kung fu or Wushu or Chinese martial arts to be the founder of the Shaolin systems of Kung fu. Modern Tai Chi is a mixture of Taoist influences, as we have seen, but also, in the physical sense, of Shaolin influences. The more obvious techniques of the Chen style of Tai Chi for instance have Shaolin roots.

But apart from techniques, the same stream which flowed through the writing of the *Tao Te Ching* was not unlike the stream coursing through Ch'an. When doing a Tai Chi form, the prevalence of change contrasts with the student's almost irrepressible desire to 'stick' to the previous movement and not prepare for the next one. The most common difficulty for a beginner is not the completion of a movement but the connecting movements. 'How do I get into the next movement?' is a universal question. Apart from mechanically learning how to do this, the student can be encouraged to 'be alive' to what he or she is doing, so that the mind does not wander, the muscles do not hold back and, though rooted, he or she floats, at the ready, never committed to the extreme of any of the movements. Though one would not say that the achievement of such a condition can be equated with enlightenment, it is in the same direction, because it tends to leave the interfering mind and habits of a lifetime behind and introduces something more real, more immediate.

2.   The Theory of Chi Kung

Chi

The effects of the Western scientific method on our views of life, and in particular on our views of humankind, have produced a one-sided outlook. Until the fairly recent past the majority of educated people looked for scientific proof before believing in a theory; at least that is what they would say if pressed. They might read their horoscopes in the daily paper but would hardly be likely to invest money in any advice they read there.

To look for scientific proof before believing some of the evidence of one's senses, and the evidence of one's experience, curtails one's view of the world. Feeling oppressed perhaps by the harness of the scientific outlook, more and more people look for other explanations of their experience, for the causes of ill-health and of unhappiness. One of these explanations is provided by the Chinese theory of Chi. Chi means internal or intrinsic energy, vitality, universal life-force. The very groping for a suitable word or expression indicates the paucity of our usual vocabulary in such areas. Even so, to use one word to explain another does not prove that the thing named exists in the first place. If we dispense with scientific, measurable, repeatable proof of the existence of something, but insist on believing in it, then common-sense says we must be able to experience its existence. If we ourselves cannot experience it just now then we can rely on first-hand accounts by reliable witnesses.

One of the major problems with the theory of Chi, from the point of view of many members of the Western medical profession for instance, is that they do not accept a direct cause and effect link in experiences where Chi is supposed to have been instrumental in bringing that experience about. For instance, it is undeniable that the insertion of acupuncture needles in certain points of the body can:

- be followed by an alleviation of pain
- be followed by a state of localized anaesthesia
- be followed by a reduction in symptoms of illness.

The important phrase here is 'be followed by'. Some Western physicians argue that it is not necessary to suppose that any unmeasurable force, called Chi, is operating in these cases. They do not all say what the cause and effect link may consist of, but they strongly affirm that Chi is an hypothesis. A detectable group of substances called endorphins act on the body to produce a calming effect. Regular, persistent, extended exercise sessions of different types have the effect of causing the body to produce endorphins. This is part of the experience of 'feeling good' after a workout or training session. Some people state that acupuncture therapy helps to stimulate endorphin production and that is the reason why it works. It has also been suggested that during hibernation animals produce a larger quantity of endorphins to enable them to endure the cold of winter.

Friends of mine returning from China, and current Chinese literature on the subject, point to the important and it seems growing role of visualization and imagination in Chi Kung, the cultivation of Chi. This gives even more strength to the argument that Chi is something which exists in or is very dependent on that murky area, 'the mind', and that 'the mind' is able to influence the state of the body if channelled in certain directions with sufficient regularity and persistence. What exactly 'the mind' is, well everyone understands that! A famous Tai Chi master in Beijing, I was told last autumn (1992), is working on visualization techniques to be done whilst performing a new Tai Chi Form which he has produced.

I do not draw any hard and fast conclusions from the above paragraphs but simply underline for readers the vagueness which exists for many Western people concerning the subject of Chi. Chinese followers of the theory of Chi, and there are many, are sure that Chi does exist. Once you accept that it does, or suspend your doubts, then a whole new universe of ideas and concepts opens up. Some of this universe is documented – carefully recorded and painstakingly pursued fact. Some of it is fantastic, or if not fantastic, theoretical in the extreme.

How Chi Kung Works

If we wish to do so we can divide Chi Kung activity into several areas, so that we have:

- medical Chi Kung
- self-development Chi Kung
- martial arts Chi Kung
- Taoist Chi Kung
- Buddhist Chi Kung
- Chi Kung connected with an art or craft
- Chi Kung connected with dance and theatrical performance
- Chi Kung for unusual feats of endurance.

In fact, it is probably true to say that in most Chinese activities which have some antiquity a form of Chi Kung exists. Chi Kung, of whatever form, takes a view of human beings which is radically different from the Western view. It is not based on the dissection and overall measurement and testing of the visible body, or the body which can be tested with electrical equipment, sounding devices and X-rays, but on a traditional picture which has been in existence for over two thousand years. This picture is based on personal experience. That is to say, that skilled and sensitive physicians, Taoist and Buddhist priests, artists and craftspeople, and others are unanimous in their assertion that the picture presented in pictorial form in Chinese manuscripts and books corresponds to the inner experience, one could almost say 'sensory' experience, which they have had. Traditional physicians claim they can sense the Chi state in a pulse or an area of the body, with their sensitive fingers. Priests state that they experience the movement of Chi within themselves, as do some martial artists. Of course, Western medical men and women can also tell a great deal about a patient from touching and 'listening' to the body.

Most of the books available on Chi Kung contain a highly simplified presentation of the subject. They are like a child's biology textbook compared with *Gray's Anatomy*. Advanced works on Chi Kung, especially the medical ones, require years of study to absorb, let alone use. Briefly, the picture of human beings used in the study of Chi Kung shows two major channels of energy. One runs down the front of the body, bisecting it, as it were, and the other runs along the back, following the middle of the spinal column. They meet just behind the sexual organs and at the roof of the mouth. At specific places on the two main channels are centres of energy collection or focus. All the organs of the body are connected through invisible channels which extend through and out on to the surface of the body. Each organ has its own specific Chi or vital energy, and when a human being is fit and well the balance between these respective energies is at its optimum. When an organ becomes deficient, Yin, in its Chi supply, or too full, Yang, physicians can detect this and using their acupuncture needles, or their fingers, or their herbs, or a combination of them, they can endeavour to redress this balance. It follows from this that each type of needle insertion, each form of finger pressure, and the chemical content of each herb is more or less Yin or Yang in relation to the condition being treated.

Chi Kung exercises aim to help an individual redress this balance or maintain this balance through his or her own efforts, so that a visit to a physician is only necessary when personal application has failed. There are many Chi Kung Forms or groups of movement sequences. Some of them involve combining breathing with movement, visualization combined with movement and breathing, and so on. Others are completely static; that is, the body itself shifts as little as possible. In the main, the remedial types of Chi Kung encourage those parts of the body, of the nervous system, which have to do with the restoring of the body to homeostasis; that is, the forces of the body which operate to maximum effect during sleep or enforced bed rest. In the ancient and modern Western medical tradition this was called *vis medicatrix naturae* – the healing power of nature. It is worth remembering that if anyone sits still for say fifteen minutes then he or she is bound to 'feel better' whether we accept the existence of Chi or not.

Moving on to other uses of Chi Kung we find that one of the energy centres which plays a major part in both martial arts and 'religious' Chi Kung is located below the navel and several centimetres inside the body. It is called in popular literature the 'tan tien'. This is a location where Chi may be accumulated, stored and released. In the case of martial artists it can be released in the form of a technique, but in the case of a Buddhist or Taoist priest it can be directed along the two main channels and through the use of meditation techniques is said to be able to assist in reaching enlightenment. Among some Taoists the use of Chi Kung was believed to lead to immortality. Whether this was literally believed or taken to be figuratively true depends on which books one reads and to whom one speaks. There is much literature on this subject. Some of it appears to be contradictory, but perhaps with sufficient study it might not prove to be so. In the current popular Chinese literature on Chi Kung the existence of a state which one would call enlightened is now admitted. A short time ago it did not correspond to the political climate. At another time it was admitted.

One of the easily verifiable phenomena accompanying Chi Kung exercise is the production of local heat, for instance in the palms of the hands. By focusing the mind on the palms they can become hot. The Chi Kung explanation for this is that the Chi is drawn to the palms, where certain major acupuncture points are located, and the excess of Chi produces heat. This experience is common among Tai Chi students. It is also said that by special exercises a Chi Kung practitioner can transmit healing Chi through his or her palms. Friends of mine say they have been helped with serious health problems by techniques such as these, used by a healer. A mother soothing an upset child by stroking is a simple example of the use of the palm. This is natural and spontaneous Chi Kung healing.

When a human being is conceived in its mother's womb it begins to receive the Chi of its parents. This is classed as 'inherited' Chi. During gestation it continues to receive the benefits of this Chi, and also Chi from the outside world in the form of air, food and drink taken in by its mother, and from any other external sources of Chi. When the child is born it begins to absorb Chi from the outside world through its own efforts. During life the effects of inherited Chi continue to be experienced and they combine with the Chi absorbed from outside and 'processed' in the body. Chi Kung is a method of regulating the Chi intake, should it have become unbalanced, insufficient, and so on. The Chi Kung of religious ways is performed not merely to prolong life and bring health but to utilize Chi to bring about a new form of experience, to realize an inherent potential for further development, and to assist the internal coordination necessary for this development.

Types of Chi Kung

Chi Kung of certain types is a form of internal alchemy or transformation of energy. In particular the Taoist school of Chi Kung left ample traces of this idea in its writings and practices. To follow this teaching requires the help of a Taoist adept, and it would be a mistake in my view to believe one could learn such things from a book, and an even bigger mistake to 'dabble' in such things out of curiosity. One can see similarities between the Taoist school and that of some schools of Yoga, Tibetan Buddhism and Sufism. Although the symbolic language used in each school is different and depends on local cultural conditions, one can assume that the aims are the same or very similar. Comparisons have also been made between the Eastern systems and the schools of early European alchemy. I refer readers to the book *In Search of the Miraculous* by P. D. Ouspensky for the best modern exposition of this type of idea which I know.

In our times the best-known forms of Chi Kung are the Eight Pieces of Brocade, Wild Goose Chi Kung and Five Animal Chi Kung. These methods have been given a definite form by people who are reputed to be experts in the field but I can neither affirm nor deny their suitability for Western people. There are as I have already said many forms of Chi Kung, and in a sense a form or laid-down method is only a door, a way in. If a form causes a student to stop searching then it has not served its purpose; so any form should be seen in this light.

The Eight Pieces of Brocade is a series of very simple movements, combined with regulated breathing and concentration, which stimulate the Chi and conduct it to various parts of the body. Compared with the other two mentioned methods it is static. Wild Goose Chi Kung consists of many relatively complicated movements, again combined with breathing, which remind one of Western calisthenics, in a sense, and the sequence of movements is much longer than the Eight Pieces of Brocade. Five Animal Chi Kung copies the movements of the bear, crane, deer, tiger and monkey. From the point of view of freedom to experiment, the Five Animals is best. This is because, although there are certain formalized movements which are the basis of the Chi Kung, there is an area in which the student relies on his or her own inspiration or inner responses. Once the basics have been learned the student may 'play' the Five Animals, and so is automatically led to search and try out variations on the basics. Proceeding in this fashion the whole experience can remain much more alive and less constricted by forms.

The 'map' of the channels or 'chinglo' of Chi energy can be found in any authentic book on acupuncture. The picture is too complex for this book. However, in Chi Kung theory there are certain points on the body which are said to be stimulated or sedated by certain types of movement. For instance, in the martial art of Hsing-I there is a point on the index finger which is said to be stimulated when the hand is clenched to make a specific type of fist formation. This point is considered to be beneficial to the lungs. My own Hsing-I teacher, Ji Jian Cheng of Hangzhou in Southern China, said that his teacher emphasized this point when he taught because he himself had found it to be helpful during his own long years of training. Dr Alexander Macdonald reported that before 1982 (precise date not given) he conducted a study of 52 patients who were experiencing pain. He found that in drawings of the pain areas and their connections the patients showed 'pain pathways' which corresponded to the chinglo paths rather than the nerve paths of Western medicine. When needles are inserted there is sometimes an impression of 'warm water' flowing along the chinglo lines. Though subjective, there is sufficient of this type of reporting for any reasonable person to grant that 'there must be something to it'.

Proviso

Chi Kung theory is based on the proposition that certain exercises, breathing methods and mental concentration can act in a similar way to the needles, though perhaps less dramatically and powerfully in the case of the majority of practitioners. Chi Kung training varies in quality from the very fine, static methods of the Taoist alchemists to the strong, muscle assisted methods of the toughest martial artists of Wushu or Kung fu. Personally I have certain provisos with regard to Chi Kung. In the first place the people who have promulgated it in the field of martial arts, from Tai Chi to Shaolin Kung fu, are on the whole much less well informed about human physiology and well-being than Chinese, or Western, physicians. Their detailed knowledge of the effects, on an individual basis, is meagre. This is not universally true but in the main it is true. Secondly, there is no regulatory body such as the British Medical Association or the General Medical Council to collate, verify and check what any individual is doing. A particular practitioner may remain isolated for years, pursuing his or her own study, with no one of comparable understanding to check and verify what is being done and perhaps passed on to students. Thus, a given practitioner can as it were go out on a limb and lose sight of many things which are necessary to safeguard individuals.

In the case of some Chinese teachers, one safeguard was the practice of taking on very few students, so that the teacher could give individual attention to each. There have been reported cases in the USA of students getting into a psycho-physical mess, due to mass tuition of Chi Kung. At the same time, this need not deter students who are capable of taking a careful, slow approach to the subject from trying it out under the guidance of a competent teacher. One other safeguard which I have always emphasized myself is to be very careful when influencing the breathing. Never try to force or mentally regulate breathing. As in the case of Tai Chi also, correct breathing will 'suggest' itself when the body is sufficiently relaxed. Having said this, one can only hope that Chi Kung will find a place for itself in current Western therapeutic methods.

3. Aspects of Physics in Tai Chi

Leaving considerations such as Chi power aside for a while, readers may find it interesting to look at some aspects of conventional physics which can be seen in the study and practice of Tai Chi. It can be argued that whatever force is used in Tai Chi, and however this force is produced, in the final analysis the force acts through laws formulated by Isaac Newton and investigated by later generations of physicists. Phenomena which by-pass the laws of physics we call miracles but if the levitation of 'yogis' and Christian saints is true, then some die-hard physicists might argue even then that they did it by an unknown means, but that that means itself really conformed to physical laws.

Three Basic Laws

All people are subject to gravity. This force is taken for granted to such an extent that we don't notice it, except indirectly when we fall or lose our balance, or ride on a swing. Yet it is always there, keeping us firmly down on the earth instead of bouncing up and down like astronauts. But if gravity is taken for granted, another force is hardly ever even acknowledged. This is the force which counters the force of gravity. For every force which acts upon us there is an equal and opposite force. The reason why we don't plunge down into the earth's core, like a deep sea diver with lead-weighted feet sinking through the ocean, is because there is a force coming up, so to speak, from the ground, balancing the force of gravity. Gravity pulls and drags us down but the other force pushes us back up. This is a difficult notion to grasp at first but if you weigh it up for a while you will see it.

According to Tai Chi, these two forces meet in the body, and near the base of the spine they 'flatten out', as it were, keeping the body stable. This region, in the abdomen, is also usually regarded both in Tai Chi and sports training as the centre of gravity. In Tai Chi the Bow Stance, described later (page 81) in the practical section of the book, ensures that a student's centre of gravity is well placed between the two legs, giving stability. If the centre of gravity is shifted so that it rests almost entirely over one leg then the posture is much less stable, because the base support is more narrow. It is also less stable because the arms, the other leg and the head and trunk have to be focused over that narrower base. With weight on one leg, the movement of an arm away from the axis, or the tilting of the head, can cause such a change in weighting that a person might fall over, as we all know.

These facts explain why in the majority of Tai Chi styles the trunk is held erect, the head 'suspended', chin sunk, elbows down, knees bent, and so on. These ways of holding and moving the body contribute to keeping a firm base and a stable posture in which the energy can circulate, without the eruption of tensions in the body aimed at maintaining balance.

A second theory from the world of physics is that if a body of whatever kind is travelling in a certain direction, it will continue to do so, unless another force is brought to bear upon it causing it to change direction. So when a Tai Chi student is moving forwards, let us say in the movement known as Ward Off Left (see page 52), his or her rear leg is propelling the trunk forwards, both feet flat on the ground. According to physics, unless another force is brought to bear the student would continue to move forward, and if the feet were not moved, the student would topple over forwards. In the case of the movement Ward Off Right, the new force enters in the shape of a turn to the right to begin Roll Back movement. The feet do not have to move because the direction of the trunk movement is changed from directly forward into a twisting movement to the right. In turn the twisting movement to the right is arrested by torsion, that is, the waist/pelvis twisting back to the left. As one movement leads into another, each force in a certain direction is countered by another force moving in a different direction. Tai Chi movements are so designed, and the way they are performed is so designed, that the change of direction of forces is relatively smooth and there is no sudden meeting of contrary forces which would result in a shock to the body; something which occurs frequently in Karate for instance.

The third 'law' of physics is that in order to produce acceleration in the movement of a body the force applied must equal the mass of the object multiplied by the acceleration. In Tai Chi the body is supposed to move at a uniform speed and in most Forms this is true. However it does happen in all the Forms with which I am familiar that there is an occasional acceleration. The most obvious cases are the movements involving spins and kicks, such as Sweep Lotus With Leg (see page 76), where the leg is swung up and across the body at a greater speed than in other parts of the Form. Additionally, there are the instances which occur involuntarily when a student speeds up during a Form due to loss of attention. What is of interest to us as Tai Chi students, here, is how this acceleration is produced rather than a precise measurement in terms used by physicists. In Sweep Lotus some insight into the production of acceleration can be found by examining just what happens before this acceleration.

What has happened is that the body has spun round on one leg from left to right through 360 degrees. Before the spin the body was in a posture called Stand on One Leg To Ride The Tiger, or Mount The Tiger (see page 75). From the Tiger position the student steps forward, at usual uniform speed, on to the right leg, *twisting* to the left, arms horizontally spread out to the sides. This twist, or torsion, to the left, provides us with a clue to the source of the additional force which provides acceleration for the spin. As the upper body turns on the waist to the left, the lower body begins to twist in the opposite direction to the right, preparing for the spin. The waist torsion, like the wringing out of a wet dish cloth, produces what is needed, and the left foot increases this force with a push to send the body spinning round on the ball of the right foot. As the body completes its spin, going into Sweep Lotus, a similar force is generated from the opposite side. Having completed its spin from right to left, the arms carry round to the right side of the body. The right leg sweeps left, up and horizontally across while the arms sweep in the opposite direction. The source of power is again coming from the torsion of the body, combined with a push from the floor by the feet.

Leaving aside all Chinese explanations in traditional writings as to how the body moves and what forces are employed, we can see that the movements of Tai Chi can be analysed in terms of these three laws in Western physics. For example, as a student's study of Tai Chi deepens, he or she will begin to appreciate not only forces which increase the direction of a movement or cause it to change, but also the forces which cause acceleration to diminish, and those which tend to maintain an original position whilst other forces at the same time tend to change it.

Take the arch of the foot. Habitual misuse of the ankle joint, tending to fall inwards, is simply a 'lazy' response to the pull of gravity. The muscles which should balance a tendency to fall inwards, or rarely, outwards, at the ankle joint are not being used efficiently. They should counter the gravitational pull down and pull up and across to bring the ankle back into the correct position. But this realignment of the ankle joint need not be complicated by trying to bring isolated muscles into play. If you stand with feet apart and take a step forward on to your right foot, sole flat, and keep your weight back on your left, you can use your ankle correctly simply by ensuring that your right leg moves in the correct direction. Simply 'point' your right knee towards the middle of the spread of your toes, shift your weight on to the right foot, and guide the knee forward in the correct line. Doing this you make use of the gravitational pull down, the force reacting to gravity by pushing up, the force of pushing from the left leg to overcome the inertia of your static position, and finally the force resisting the push from your left leg which stops you losing balance and, in theory, flying forwards on to your face!

Conclusion

If you try to become aware of these forces in operation, you will probably not succeed at once. But you *will* become much more aware of what you are doing, and also *know* what you are doing, much better. Take another and more simple example. Raise your right arm in front of your shoulder, palm up and elbow slightly bent. Gravity pulls down on your arm and your muscles keep the arm up. You try to be aware of this. *Let* your arm go slowly down towards the outside of your right hip. In doing so you give way to gravity by diminishing the force which is acting against it. If you were to let your arm drop, gravity would see to it that it did drop, combining with the momentum of the mass of your arm. But instead you let it down slowly. When it is down by the side of your leg you raise it sideways, overcoming gravity again by using more force.

Notice that as you lower and raise your arm you do not stop moving. Thus, as you change the direction of the movement you are introducing additional force; force which changes the direction of movement. Though usually we do this without noticing, we are 'obeying' the law of physics which says that no object changes its direction without the application of another force powerful enough to achieve this change. If you try to be aware of these forces and changes your Tai Chi movement will improve.

4. Principles of Tai Chi Chuan

This chapter develops what was said in the previous one, about Tai Chi and physics. If we look at Tai Chi from a Western scientific point of view, interpreting the word 'scientific' to mean something which can be experimentally verified and not merely something popularly held to be true, then the principles on which Tai Chi is based can be summarised as the same principles which we find in the natural world:

No object moves or changes its direction without the application of another force.

To every force which is applied to an object there is an equal and opposite reacting force.

To produce an acceleration in the movement of a body the force applied must equal the mass of the object multiplied by the acceleration.

You will recall, perhaps, from school lessons in physics/mechanics that the above principles are a free interpretation of Newton's laws of motion. What Tai Chi does or tries to do for its followers is to enable them to experience the reality of conventional scientific principles in their movements. This is not a dry, academic enterprise, in which we struggle with concepts which seem to clog up the brain of anyone who does not find mechanics easy. On the contrary, it is not essentially an intellectual operation; but rather one in which the stark principles of Western science find their expression in an Eastern mode of movement. For, in terms of movement, what are the implications of trying to move according to the laws of physics? They imply movement in which;

1. Just the right amount of force is used to bring about a result, no more, no less;

2. No movement is made unless it is called for, no extraneous movements, no movements which go against the structure of the body;
3. An attempt to be in regular, if not constant, touch with the experience of the pull of gravity; and
4. A corresponding and simultaneous awareness of the counter-force from the ground, which is constantly being exerted against the pull of gravity.

The last point is probably the most important and, as far as I know from my own reading, it is the one which is never mentioned in Tai Chi; though it is implied in Tai Chi instruction and books. In case readers instantly pick up their pens and start writing to me care of the publishers, Element Books, I should say again that this force coming from the ground is implied in Tai Chi writings but not much, if anything, is made of it. It needs to be emphasized, and will be, in this chapter.

1. The Application of Force

Beginning with the first principle, we find in Tai Chi a saying that if a leaf were placed in the hand of a Tai Chi expert that hand would sink lower, such is the balance and optimum use of force being applied to keep that hand in place. The weight of a leaf would cause it to move, like a well-balanced pair of scales. Add a gramme weight and one side sinks. This applies to the whole body. The aim in Tai Chi is to have a body which is so balanced, with tensions and relaxations so evenly spread, that even a leaf would displace the position of the whole body.

Of course, this is an ideal, something which rarely if ever happens in humans, although fully expressed in the rest of the living world. In terms of Chinese philosophy, it is an expression of Yin and Yang balance. In Tai Chi there should be not too much Yin, yielding, softness, and not too much Yang, aggression, hardness.

2. The Balanced Body

The second principle follows from the first. The body is constructed in a particular way. The lower half, from say the top sacral vertebra, should support the rest. The lower half, responding to and at the same time equally resisting the pull of gravity, should be Yang, firm, solid, rooted. The upper half, supported by the lower, should be Yin, soft, pliable, rising or floating upward. Key areas such as the head and neck, shoulders and arms, should be especially watched so that they in a sense rise or float. The body's centre of gravity, in the lower abdomen, below the navel, including the corresponding point on the spinal column, should be the meeting place for the upper and lower parts of the body where forces are focused.

Since people who take up Tai Chi are only human, and have long since left the innocence and spontaneity of infancy behind, and with it the natural ability of the child to do Tai Chi as it were naturally, we have to take the physical condition in which we find them into account. So, for instance, almost every civilized man and woman holds his or her shoulders up, through tension. Thus, the principle of allowing the shoulders to float has no meaning for such a person, at the beginning. On the contrary, the instruction given here is for him or her to let the shoulders go down. If this is achieved and the study of Tai Chi pursued then in time the shoulders can be encouraged to float.

This example is but one of several apparent contradictions in the principles of Tai Chi which a beginner encounters. Another example concerns the tension found in civilized people in the lower back, around the back of the waist or small of the back. Before one can think of the lower part of the body supporting the upper, this tension needs to be investigated in the sense that it needs to be felt and ways of letting it go explored. It is only when the upper and lower parts, usually 'fused' into one through tension in the small of the back, are freed from one another that they can be rejoined with optimum muscle tone.

3. Being Aware of Gravity

The third principle of being in touch with the experience of gravity is part of the psychological problem of being civilized. What we call being civilized, the condition, implies an over-active, associating, 'thinking' brain and a body whose very existence we are hardly aware of unless hungry, sleepy, in need of sexual satisfaction or in pain. So the first step will be to become more aware of the body, any part of it, and in time also aware of the gravitational pull on it; one could say becoming aware of one's own body weight. The fact that a living organism has to return to an awareness of something which should be a constant in its life, through the intervention of an exercise, is something remarkable in itself.

This third principle is clearly intimately connected with the other two, preceding ones. If it were possible for us to be aware, throughout the body, of the action of gravity, and let the body respond to it, without interference, then we would not need Tai Chi, or anything like it. Partly through having an overactive brain, our awareness of gravity has been blanked out, as though certain nerve pathways in our nervous system had been severed, or at least, anaesthetized, put to sleep. By beginning to return to this awareness, to awaken and reactivate the pathways, again and again, we shall approach more of a wholeness in ourselves. Another consequence of a growing awareness of gravity, combined with the effects of exploring the other principles of Tai Chi, is that breathing may become more natural, and less impeded by unnatural tensions.

4. Using the Force from the Ground

The fourth principle, of taking in the force from the ground which counterbalances the pull of gravity, accompanies the growth of awareness of gravity. If this force did not exist, we should be pulled down through the earth to its very centre, and all be piled up on top of one another like an immense sack of human potatoes! When you think about it, the floor is exerting a force of resistance which is transmitted to the body. The feet, legs, pelvis and spine conduct this force upwards, as well as conducting the force of gravity downwards. What we could call a right conducting of these two forces produces or could produce an optimum condition like a man or woman comfortably floating in water, and simply called upon to make small adjustments to remain vertical in the water, and not tip over.

As was said before, all this is a question of principles whose optimum expression is an ideal, something to be looked towards and not something readily available. Beginning to study Tai Chi in a practical way is one approach to such an expression.

5. Introductory Exercises

Some people skip introductory exercises when they are learning something new. If exercises are included in any type of course, remember there may be a good reason for them. There is a good reason for the ones presented in this chapter so do not skip them.

As you study Tai Chi you will discover many things about yourself if you are alert. You will find that you are not aware of your habitual body posture, the line of your back, the position of your shoulders in relation to your back, neck and head, and other things which you generally take for granted. In addition, and in a sense more importantly, you will realize how tense you usually are, even if you think that you are a relaxed sort of person. Tai Chi can improve your appearance; that is, your carriage, the way you hold yourself. The following exercises will help you in this discovery and will contribute to your performance of the Tai Chi Forms and Sets as well.

Try to be patient. Water dripping down gradually wears away stone. Metal can quickly crack and shatter stone. As you are dealing with your own body, nervous system and brain, it is better to be like water. This advice might have been taken from a Taoist text and as such it fits in well with Tai Chi training. This is because Tai Chi, like Taoism and other traditional teachings, depends greatly on the development of awareness. You begin with more gross aspects such as the relative position of hands, feet, head and trunk and move on to more subtle things such as awareness of muscle tension, weight and speed and later perhaps to awareness of energy. If you try to be aware of energy immediately you will ignore the important question of correct posture and movement, which in Tai Chi should come first. You will use tension instead of relaxation to achieve results, and later if you want to deepen your Tai Chi you will have to unlearn all your bad habits. This can take a long time.

Please proceed with care when exercising; take your physical condition into account.

Exercise 1

Find a wall which has no skirting board to it and stand with your back to the wall. Both your heels touch the wall and you stand up in your habitual upright posture. Your buttocks and upper back also touch the wall. Put your hand round to the small of your back and feel the gap, which there will almost certainly be, between that region of the back and the wall. Gently push the small of the back towards the wall so that it is as flat as possible, without using force. Spend some time studying this. As you push the small of your back to the wall, try to find the most relaxed way of doing it. If you notice that you tense your abdominal muscles then bend your knees a little and try to relax your abdomen. You *let* your abdominal muscles go and *let* the back move to the wall. It is very different from forcing your body to do something. Be prepared to be patient and perhaps unsuccessful at the first few attempts.

Then, still keeping the small of the back in the same position, that is in line with the rest of the back, walk away from the wall using small steps. The purpose of this exercise is to begin a movement away from the usual over-arched small of the back which most people have. If your back is already well aligned, then ignore this exercise. It is not a question of having an unnaturally straight back, but having a more pliable back in this region of the spine. Study this change of posture and begin to notice how the change in one area affects other areas. In this way your body is allowed to become more mobile, which it is designed to be after all.

Exercise 2

Get a stick which is not more than half an inch (1 centimetre) thick and about 3 feet (1 metre) long. The section shape does not matter. Hold the stick in one hand some 4 inches (10 centimetres) from the top between your thumb and the first two fingers so that it hangs down straight in front of you. Raise and lower the stick freely, moving it about 6 inches (15 centimetres) vertically upwards and then downwards as if you were bouncing it on the floor, but it does not touch the floor. Try to feel that the stick is very free in your grip, holding very lightly, and the part of the stick below your grip hangs down; feel its weight, however small. As you do this, put the fingers of your free hand on your occiput – the point where the top of the spine meets the back base of the skull.

Use your imagination to feel that your occiput corresponds to that point of the stick which you are gripping, and that the part of the stick which is below your grip corresponds to your body below the occiput. Transfer the feeling of free movement, and 'hanging down', which is in the feeling of the stick, into your body. Bounce your body, at the knees, freely and gently, in time with the rhythm of the stick bounce. Your body 'hangs down' from the occiput. The feeling includes your shoulders, which also hang down. Then try walking and very, very slightly 'bouncing', being aware of the stick, your point of grip, your occiput and the body below it. Then take your fingers away from your head and feel the occipital region without their help.

This may result in a much greater feeling of freedom in the body, if you practise. When you think you can, add to this exercise. Allow your jaw/chin to sink down a little way, to help release tension in the back of the neck, and imagine that your head is suspended from above 'as if by a single hair', to quote an old Tai Chi saying (although these are not traditional Tai Chi exercises but simply methods developed by me or learned by me over the years).

It is not advisable to do this exercise in full view of the general public; they may have doubts about your state of mind!

Once you think you can, try also turning your head from side to side as you walk and bounce so that your head moves freely at the occiput.

These first two exercises can do much to 'set you up' for Tai Chi. Later, when you are doing the Forms, occasionally remember the two exercises, and the sense of freedom they can bring. They could help you to perform Tai Chi movements better.

Exercise 3

Stand up straight, with arms hanging down at the sides. Turn your head to the right and raise your right arm, palm up, so that it extends horizontally to your right side and you look at the palm. Bend your arm at the elbow, like a traffic policeman, and bring the palm towards your face, across the top right front of your chest and down in a curve past the lower left side of your chest, down across your groin and back up to the side. Same with the left arm. Follow the movement of the palm with your eyes/head.

Move slowly and smoothly, head and arm at the same speed. When you are confident about this, do both arms at once. That is, as soon as the right arm bends inwards from the horizontal position, start to raise the left up to the horizontal position. Turn your head left and right in harmony with the movement of the right arm. As the right arm descends begin to bend the left arm, and as the right arm begins to rise the left arm descends. Then the cycle begins again. Though perhaps tricky at first this exercise will prepare you for the Tai Chi Forms.

Once you have absorbed the movement of the two arms and head, then add the waist turn. That is to say, when your right arm rises and extends you turn your body to the right, feet remaining still, and when the right arm bends and comes in your body turns to the left. There will therefore be one turn right and one turn left for each cycle of the right arm. Alternate by beginning with the left arm. This is a movement characteristic of Tai Chi Form movements. If you become proficient at it, and others like it, then when you begin the Forms you will not find them as difficult as many people who have not had such a preparation.

To my knowledge, no one has taken the trouble to set down or even use such exercises before. They may be used in a cursory fashion by way of illustration, in a class, but that is not the same as making a definite grouping of such exercises as is being made in this book. Since all the exercises presented come from experience and not merely copying what exists, and since they have been used in teaching Western people, they should benefit the majority of English-speaking readers.

Exercise 4

In Tai Chi the position or shape taken by the palms and fingers is not to be ignored. The hands are, as it were, the completion of the Forms. If the trunk, legs, arms and head are in the correct position then the hands round off the entire shape. Perhaps because we take our hands for granted we tend to ignore the finer points of their position. If we say that the hands also have a posture or shape, even though they are small, this may help to clarify what I am saying.

Look at one of your palms. If you cup your hand a little, bringing fingers, thumb and edges of the palm inwards, you will see a central region, in which for instance you could carry a small pool of water. Chi Kung theory states that Chi can concentrate in this region. When we extend the arm, pushing the palm forwards, in Tai Chi, the Chi can sometimes be experienced moving into that part. If you do not want to use the concept of Chi then you could say that you are aware of energy in that part of the hand. The expression 'healing palms' is connected to this.

When the hands are used for pushing forward, circling, brushing, drawing back and so on in Tai Chi this central cupping of the palm should be observed so that a feeling of being related to the centre of the palms is preserved. Thus the shape and energy go hand in hand, so to speak. Then as an exercise, raise one palm in the way you would do if you were gesturing someone to stop coming towards you, or like a traffic controller, and then bring the palm into a more rounded shape, curving the fingers a little and bending the thumb slightly forward. Maintain this shape and sweep the palm round in big circles in a variety of directions, sometimes slowly rotating the wrist. When you feel happy about this, do the same thing with both palms, maintaining feeling in them, especially in the central region.

Return to the previous exercise and repeat it with the palms in this shape.

These four exercises give you some important pointers to the performance of Tai Chi Forms. The head should be free, the trunk erect with sacrum lowered (not tucked forward which causes tension) the shoulders weighed down by their own weight, and the hands given a shape.

Exercise 5

Stand with your feet apart, just wider than the width of your hips, knees bent. Slowly turn the left hip back and the right hip forward, then left hip forward and right hip back. Keep your shoulders and chest as still as you can without undue tension. Explore this hip movement and on a daily basis try to improve the freedom of movement. Next, include the whole torso in the turn so that hip and shoulder turn together. Do not raise your shoulders; keep them relaxed and down.

Bring the right palm in front of the right armpit, facing away from the body and as you turn your right hip forward let your palm push ahead, away from your right shoulder until your arm is almost, but not completely, straight. Work at this until you feel that the turning action of the trunk is sending the palm out rather than the muscles of the upper arm. Turn the palm round so that it is facing upwards, and begin to turn your torso in the opposite direction, drawing the upraised, cupped palm down in an arc towards your right hip and back beyond your right shoulder. Then lift it up in an arc towards your right shoulder and as you turn your torso you once again push the palm forwards. Do this with the left palm and afterwards combine the two. This means that as your right hip and shoulder turn to the front and your palm goes ahead your left palm will go back and down, and vice versa.

With a little application you will soon be able to perform a smooth movement, brought about mainly by the action of the turning of your waist, accompanied by contrary motion of the palms. If you compare this exercise with exercise 3, you will see that this one, though more is involved, is similar to the other. In Tai Chi the turning of the trunk is an almost constant factor, and one which largely contributes to the health and longevity Tai Chi seems to confer. A noticeable feature of the physical condition of many elderly people is that they find turning the trunk, shoulders, neck and head very difficult. Regular training in Tai Chi can help to prevent this and even remedy it.

Exercise 6

This next exercise is described in more detail in my book, *Animal Forms of Chi Kung*, but it is a useful one for Tai Chi students and I include it in outline here. It is part of the Crane series of movements.

Stand with feet close together to form a concentrated base and raise your heels several times, going up on to the balls of your feet. Then place both palms against your thighs and begin. As you raise your heels, raise both arms, palms facing downward, wrists almost straight, at an angle of 45 degrees – that is, 45 degrees to an angle formed by an arm raised straight in front. Keep the arms slightly bent, imagining that your arms are the wings of a Crane, and the curve from shoulder to index fingertip is the bony cartilage from which the feathers descend. You raise your arms, as you raise your heels, to shoulder height, then 'beat' down, slowly, to 'fly', leading with your elbows and letting forearm and palms follow. As you beat down, lower your heels and bend your knees deeply, then rise and raise your arms once again. Explore this exercise, breathing freely and letting the air circulate without forcing. Do not exaggerate the knee bend at first, until you know how much bending your knees can tolerate.

This exercise will show you something about opening the shoulders, letting the shoulders work and giving them more freedom. If your arms and shoulders ache it is because you are too tense. Try to find out how much force you need and do not use more than that, unless you choose to do so.

Exercise 7

A dozen or more muscles and tendons are attached to the scapula, or shoulder blade; it also forms a joint at the top of the shoulder with the collar bone. You can touch the scapula by putting your left hand over your right shoulder and feeling for an almost horizontal bony ridge just below the ridge of the shoulder muscles. You can also push the back of your left palm up the right side of your trunk and feel a triangular, mobile, bony area which moves over your rib cage at the back when you move your arms. This amazing piece of 'machinery' helps the arm to remain in place when it moves in the shoulder socket. Since it would be very difficult to seek out and relax all the muscles attached to the scapula we can say that one tries to 'relax the scapula'. As it is bone and gristle it does not relax in the same way as a muscle, but this formulation or instruction gives you a focus and it works.

When you push your right palm forward in front of your shoulder you try keeping the flat of the back of your left palm on the scapula. When you have pushed as far forward as you can comfortably do, extend the arm even further forward and you will feel the scapula contribute to the extension. So try gently circling the shoulder up, forward, down and back, and so forth, concentrating on the scapula movement; relax it, become aware of it – and your shoulders and arms will relax.

I received a letter from an elderly lady some years ago. She had heard of this exercise using the scapula and with its help she relaxed her shoulders to such an extent that she was able to give up taking painkilling medication prescribed for her shoulder pains. As she had been learning Tai Chi from a Chinese teacher for several years before learning of my exercise it made me wonder just what had been happening in her classes. In any case the exercise is recommended. It too will help you with Tai Chi Forms.

It is worth bearing in mind that whilst exercise is not a substitute for medical treatment, from whatever source, it does have the merit of being cheaper – it's free! The more you understand your own body, through training, the more you will increase your capacity to take care of yourself. There must be millions of people complaining of some ache or pain in their bodies which is caused either by immobility or regular misuse. Tai Chi is one of the methods which can help this: a preventive therapy. Another of my students, a middle-aged woman, came to a class one day with very bad back pain. She said that she thought she would not be able to join in but would try. I toned all the exercises down, doing very gentle Chi Kung and she did join in. In the afternoon of that same day her back pain had gone. This might have been pure coincidence but perhaps not.

Exercise 8

Rub the palms of both hands together for a while until you begin to feel heat in them. This is a simple device to warm up the hands and, as Chi Kung students would say, to bring Yang energy to them. Put both palms on the top of your head and firmly stroke down over your face, neck and chest to the lower abdomen. Begin again from the head and stroke down the sides of the head, sides of the chest and into the abdomen. Put your palms at the back of your head and stroke down the back of the neck, over the shoulders and down the front of the chest to the abdomen. Place the palms as high up the back as you comfortably can, on either side of the spine, and stroke down, over your kidneys and buttocks and up over the hip joints back to the abdomen. Occasionally rub the palms again to warm them up.

Put your palms on the buttocks and stroke down the backs of the legs to the heels. Stroke down the sides, front and insides of the legs. Some students find this stroking, firmly, very restorative. You stroke *down* to bring the fire, the warmth, the Yang, downwards, away from the head and heart, which, in figurative language, should be cool. When fire is in the head there is confusion and when too much fire is in the heart the pulse is agitated. Whatever your opinion concerning this type of terminology, try the exercise and, if you benefit and it has no ill-effects, then use it.

Exercise 9

Lastly, pay attention to the eyes. In Tai Chi the eyes and head follow the leading direction; that is, the direction of the Form, which often means the direction in which the body weight is moving. Practise keeping your head still and without force turn your eyes from left to right, up and down, diagonally up and down and then rotate them. Then do the same and let your head *follow*. Your aim in fact is to move eyes and head *together*, but the feeling is that the eyes are in a sense leading the movement. Do not strain or stare. Then try moving one of your palms about in different directions, and follow the palm with your eyes/head. Then try moving your eyes/head in different directions and follow that direction with your palm. You will find the two experiences quite different. An onlooker would probably not be able to tell the difference but you will be able to do so.

When you come to do the Tai Chi Forms later, do not think about the eyes. You will have enough on your plate without bringing the eyes into it. But if you have some awareness of the eyes, at the back of your mind as it were, then this will help. The eyes, like the hands, are often taken for granted.

6. Learning the 48 Form Set of Tai Chi

In some Chinese martial arts traditions, a student always faces south when beginning to do a Form. This is because the south is the bringer of warmth and good fortune. You may feel you wish to follow this tradition. In any case it is good to begin always in the same place, facing the same direction, since this helps you to remember the movements. If you train outdoors you begin to associate, say, the garden wall or the sycamore tree with a particular movement. This is my experience. However, once you have 'got' the Form it will not matter where you stand. In describing the movements of this sequence we shall use the Western clock face, 1 to 12, to locate them. You imagine yourself standing in the centre of a horizontal clock.

During the 1920s, Chinese army officers and politicians combined with a number of famous martial artists to found centres of martial arts training. The stated aim of these centres was to improve the fitness and morale of troops, and foster health, strength and fitness in the nation. This move brought about contacts between martial arts teachers and experts which might not have otherwise taken place. It gave an impetus to training and a focus. Some of the men and women who were influenced by these centres survived the Japanese invasion of China, the turmoil of the Revolution and the hectic years of the post-revolutionary period. In turn they influenced the decisions of the State Commission for Physical Culture and Sports in China who produced what is called the Simplified Form of Taiji (Tai Chi) or 24 Step (Forms) Beijing (Peking) Form of Taiji, during the 1950s. This Form is mainly an off-shoot of Yang-style Tai Chi. A video and book in English was produced on the Form, and it had wide popularity. In a sense this Form is easy, if any Tai Chi can be said to be easy; it is also relatively short; in any event the demand for something more testing, some longer Form, was satisfied by the 48 Step, or 48 Forms, of Taiji, also born in the 1950s.

The question of translations haunts martial arts literature, and the use of the word 'Step' only really makes sense if you think of it as 'steps to be taken', in the sense of 'what you must do to'. So a translation would read: 'the 24 steps (Forms of movement you must do)'. Unfortunately, for universal clarity, Western people have become accustomed to calling the whole sequence of movements a Form. Chinese books translated into English have called each separate group of movements a Form, and have called the whole sequence of movements a Set. Ergo, a Set consists in this instance of 48 Forms. It seems preferable to fall in with the Chinese translators to preserve some uniformity in describing the movements here. Even so I prefer the older Western usage. A custom which confuses the issue even more is the Western translation of each separate group of movements of the Set by the word Posture. This is because there are in each Set a number of positions which can be taken and held, statically, for training purposes and purposes of Chi Kung. When the Set is performed, these positions or Postures are never held and so cannot accurately be called Posture. What the Chinese mean by a Form is those movements which are done between one Posture and another and the final position of each movement. Thus:

> **Form** – the most widespread Western term for the whole movement series
> **Form** – the Chinese translation for each separate, named, movement
> **Posture** – the Western term for the different statically taken positions
> **Set** – the Chinese translation for the whole movement series.

When reading or listening you just need to be clear in which sense the words are being used.

One more word about translation. If you are familiar with some of the old Tai Chi Forms you will notice some differences in terminology. The two most notable examples are Step Back and Whirl Arms (Step Back to Drive Monkey

Away) and Fan Penetrates Back (Flash the Arm). Obviously the Chinese translators did not know the naked significance of flashing!

Below is a list of movements in the Set; these are each covered in detail, in the same order, later in this chapter. Some movements are repeated; probably because their exercise, martial and Chi Kung significance is considered more important. For instance the movement called Grasp the Sparrow's Tail is repeated several times to stimulate the Chi in a particular manner. Consequently, there are not 48 different movements or Forms, but 48 Forms.

Preparation and Beginning
White Crane Spreads Wings
Brush Left Knee and Twist
Left Single Whip
Play Guitar (Lute) Left
Stroke and Push
Strike, Parry and Punch Left
Ward Off, Roll Back, Press and Push Left
Diagonal Leaning
Punch Under Elbow
Step Back and Whirl Arms (Step Back to Drive Monkey Away)
Turn and Push
Play Guitar (Lute) Right
Brush Knee and Punch Down
White Snake Puts Out Tongue
Pat Foot to Tame Tiger
Turn Left and Strike
Threading Palm and Crouch Down
Ward Off Standing On One Leg
Right Single Whip
Wave Hands Like Clouds
Part Wild Horse Mane
High Pat On Horse
Kick With Right Heel
Strike With Both Fists
Kick With Left Heel
Punch With Concealed Fist
Needle At Sea Bottom
Fan Penetrates Back (Flash the Arm)
Kick With Right and Left Feet
Brush Left and Right Knees
Step Up and Punch
As if Closing a Door

Wave Hands Like Clouds
Turn Right and Strike
Fair Lady Works With Shuttles
Step Back With Cross-over Palm
Press Down Palms With Empty Step
Stand On One Leg Holding Out Palm
Push Forearm With Horse Stance
Turn Body With Large Strokes
Swinging Palms and Crouching Step (Single Whip Squat-ting Down)
Step Up and Cross Fists
Stand On One Leg to Ride the Tiger
Sweep Lotus With Leg
Bend the Bow to Shoot the Tiger
Strike, Parry and Punch
Ward Off, Roll Back, Press and Push Right
Crossing Hands
Closing.

When you see other people doing this Set proficiently you will observe two broad categories of performance. One will be those people who have learned from a good teacher, and they will reproduce it as accurately as they can. The other will be those people who have learned accurately and who have absorbed the Set into their own way of doing Tai Chi. The latter's performance will be influenced by such things as the effects of learning the older Yang style, or Chen style or Wu style; the result of Chi Kung, Pa Kua Chang or Hsing-I training; or a mixture of these. As much as a book can, given the space available and the limits of the written word, the following descriptions give an accurate account of the way the Set is done in China today. From time to time changes to a Set are made. Such changes are usually small.

Preparation and Beginning

Stand as in Figure 1 facing towards 12 on an imaginary clock. You are relaxed and alert. Pause for as long as you wish, so that you can concentrate on the matter in hand and forget about everything else. When you are ready, raise the left heel until the toes alone are on the ground, then place it flat down, toe first, the width of your hips away from your right foot, so that both feet are parallel to one another; both flat on the floor. As you take this small step, rotate both arms in their shoulder sockets, a little, so that your palms face behind you, to 6 on the clock, your elbows bend slightly and both knees bend a little. All the movements should be slow and synchronized.

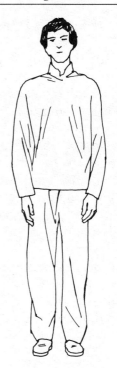

Fig. 1

Once you start to move, you move at the same speed throughout the Set. You never stop moving until the end. Then bring your arms forward and upward as high as your shoulders, elbows bent a little outwards and wrists forming a continuous curve between hand and arm. Fingers are spread a little and palms hollowed (Figure 2).

Lower your elbows bringing them in towards your lower ribs and let the hands follow simply, then press the palms down level with the navel. Simultaneously with the descent of the arms, bend your knees a little more. If the bent knee position is too hard on your knees then 'stand high'; that is, bend your knees only marginally.

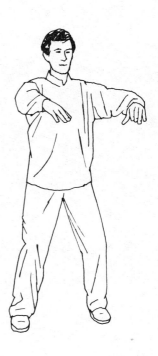

Fig. 2

White Crane Spreads Wings

Turn your body a little to the left, shifting your weight on to the left leg. As you do this, bring your left palm up in front of your left shoulder, about the same distance from it as the length of your upper arm, and bring your right arm across your body so that it is under your left palm, waist level, as if holding a ball with both hands (Figure 3). Bring your right foot close to the instep of your left foot, heel raised and look in the direction of your left hand.

Move your right foot backwards and a little outwards and shift your weight on to it, turning your body to the right, bringing your right arm, palm vertical and facing inwards, across to the right, head height, and lowering the left palm, downward facing, so that the fingers are pointing towards the right elbow (Figure 4). Raise the heel of your left foot.

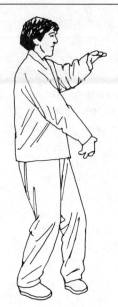

Fig. 3

Complete this Form by 'brushing' the left palm across the front of your body, fingers pointing to the front, raising the right palm a little higher, and bringing it closer to your head, palm inwards (Figure 5).

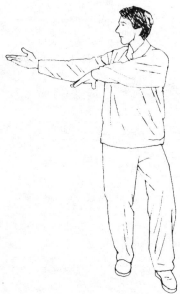

Fig. 4

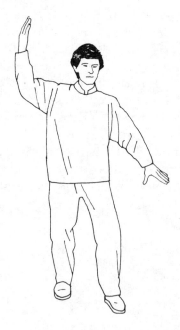

Fig. 5

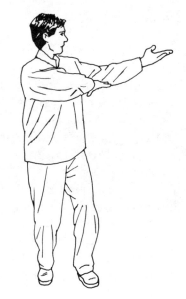

Fig. 6

Brush Left Knee and Twist

Turn the body a little left, raising the left arm, palm in, level with the face, and lowering the right arm, palm passing face and breastbone. Turn the body right, bringing left foot, heel raised, close to right instep, right palm continuing to circle down past right hip and up as high as face, palm in, while left palm crosses in front of chin and descends to a position opposite right ribs (Figures 6 and 7).

Turn the body towards the front once again, 12 o'clock, stepping with left foot towards 11 o'clock, push forward with the right hand, past your right ear and out in front of your face as you 'brush' down in front of your left knee with your left palm downward facing, fingers front (Figure 8).

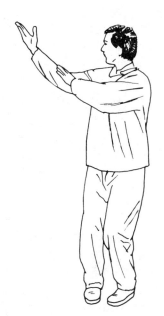

Fig. 7

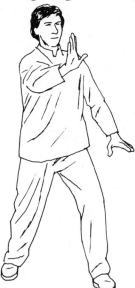

Fig. 8

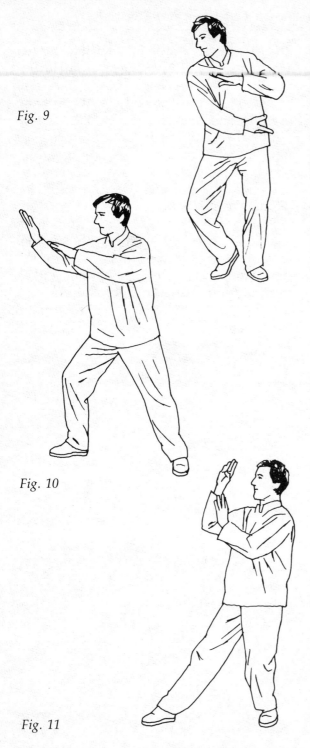

Fig. 9

Fig. 10

Fig. 11

Left Single Whip

Shift body weight firmly on to the right leg, bending the knee and raising the toes of the left foot, turning the body to the right; simultaneously let the right arm, palm down, move out to the right with the body turn and bring the left palm forward, upward and round to the right level with the left shoulder.

Replace toes of left foot on the ground and shift body weight on to that foot, then place right foot beside the left heel, toes only touching the ground and pointing away at right angles to the left heel. As the body changes position the right arm bends at the elbow, palm up and under the left elbow (Figure 9).

Now step towards 3 on the clock face with the right foot and shift the weight on to it. As you begin this step gently place the left fingertips just below the right wrist. As you shift your weight on to the right leg move both hands, still touching, in a soft curve from left towards right round to 3 (Figure 10).

Continue this sequence by shifting weight back on to the left leg, knee bending, and raise the right toes. Turn the body a little to the right and with hand/wrist still touching curve the palms out to 4 then 5 then 6 on the clock through a horizontal arc (Figure 11). (This movement is similar to a movement of the Pa Kua Chang Swimming Dragon Form (Set). It reminds us that these modern Sets are composites or syntheses of older Sets.)

Turn the body back towards 12 or 1, likewise the right foot turns in the same direction, sole flat on floor, and left heel is raised. As you do this bend the right wrist down smoothly, bringing all fingers and thumb together in a hook or beak, and push the beak out towards 3; left palm turns upward (Figure 12).

Turn the body left and step out with the left foot towards 9 on the clock. Shift weight on to the left foot, keep the right arm with the beak outstretched and slightly bent at the elbow, and bring the left palm, turned towards the body, past the nose and left shoulder, and push it out towards 9 (Figure 13).

Play Guitar (Lute) Left

Bring your right foot forward a few inches to place the toes behind and to the left of the left foot, opening the right hook hand to travel round in a horizontal arc, elbow almost straight, ahead of the right shoulder as you press down in front of you with the left palm to waist level.

Lower the right heel so foot is flat and, putting your weight on it, squat down on the right leg, almost straightening the left leg and placing the left heel, only, on the ground; your right palm circles out and down in front of your waist and your left palm circles up and forward so that you end in a position similar to that of playing a guitar, or lute (Figure 14).

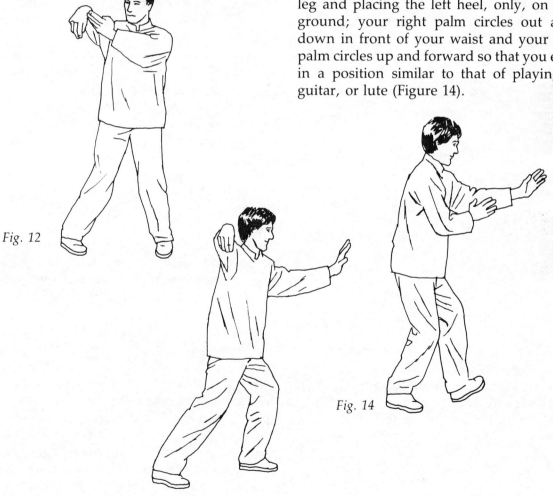

Fig. 12

Fig. 13

Fig. 14

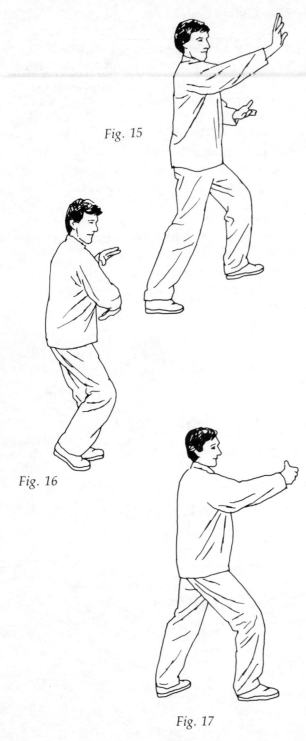

Fig. 15

Fig. 16

Fig. 17

Stroke and Push

Lower the left hand and raise the right as if pushing someone away to your right front corner, stepping to your left front corner with your left leg and shifting your weight on to it. Your body turns to face in the same direction as your right hand and the left palm also faces in this direction (Figure 15).

Both arms and the right foot move together: stroke down towards your body with both palms, your left coming to your left hip and your right in front of your abdomen; right foot steps beside left foot, heel raised (Figure 16).

Bring your right arm up in front of your chest and 'point' the fingers of the left hand towards the right forearm, stepping with your right heel towards 10 on the clock face. The movement continues with a shifting of the weight on to the right foot. (This movement is similar to the Ward Off Right of Yang style.) (Figure 17.)

Shift weight backwards once more on to left leg raising right toes, then return weight to right leg, lowering toes; at the same time, slide the left palm over the right forearm and push out the left palm as if pushing someone away from you, cupping the right palm below and back from the left elbow.

You then repeat the movement on the left side by stroking down to your right hip with your right hand and to the abdomen with your left, the left foot stepping beside the right foot, heel raised. Left arm comes up in front of your chest and right fingers 'point' at left forearm; left foot steps towards 8 on the clock, heel only, then shift weight on to left foot. Repeat on the right side shifting the weight on to the right leg, raising left heel, sliding right palm over left forearm and shifting weight back on to left leg and pushing out with vertical right palm with left palm below right elbow and back from it. Stroke down with both hands bringing right foot close to left, heel raised, then step out with right foot towards 10 raising right hand in front of chest and pointing left fingers at forearm.

Strike, Parry and Punch Left

(You will have noticed by now that in Tai Chi Forms the weight is shifted back, almost always, before another movement is made. Begin to anticipate this and it will help you to learn. A saying which I coined years ago for my own students is: 'When in doubt, shift your weight'.)

So, shift weight on to the left leg, drawing the right palm, upward facing, to the right hip in a downward curve, stretching the left arm out ahead, palm facing away from the body, raising right toes (Figure 18).

Continue to circle the right palm obliquely back and outwards, bending the elbow so that the palm comes to rest ahead of the right shoulder, downward facing; at the same time lower the left hand in a fist to the right lower ribs, palm down; weight is shifted on to the right foot and the left foot joins it, heel raised (Figure 19).

Press down to the right hip with the right palm, striking forwards and downwards with the left fist, backhand, bringing the left heel down with the leg almost straight, more or less in line with the left arm (Figure 20).

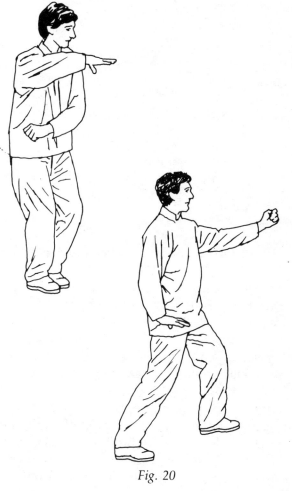

Fig. 19

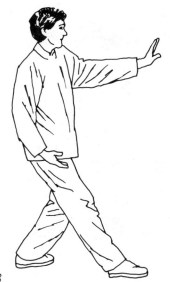

Fig. 18

Fig. 20

Shift weight on to the left foot, and step forwards with the right foot, heel only on the ground, bringing the left fist back to waist level and the right palm round in a swinging action, and forwards, as if to push aside a punch.

Shift weight on to the right leg, punching forwards with the left fist, vertically held, bringing the right palm beside the left forearm, inwards facing (Figure 21).

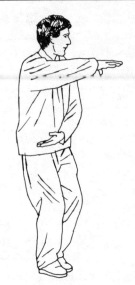

Fig. 22

Step forward with left foot, shifting weight on to it, knee bent, raising left arm ahead of chin, palm facing chin, almost straight, pressing down to hip level with right palm (Figure 23).

Turn body a little to the left so it is facing forwards, 9 on clock, thrusting forwards at hip level with right palm, upward facing, and turning left palm in a small circle so that palm faces away from chin.

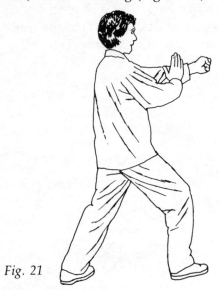

Fig. 21

Ward Off, Roll Back, Press and Push Left

Weight shifts to left leg, toes of right foot are lifted and body turns right as left palm opens to push a few inches (5–10 centimetres) across to the right and right palm descends upward facing to right hip.

Weight shifts to right foot, flat, and left foot steps slightly ahead and to side of right, toes touching only, as left palm descends, upward facing in front of waist and right circles back then forward to rest at chin level above left, as if holding a ball (Figure 22). Just like Figure 19 but lower palm open.

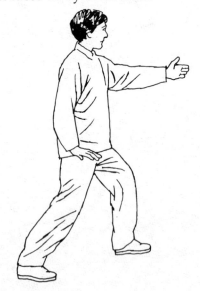

Fig. 23

Weight shifts back on to right leg, both palms stroke downwards (Figure 24), past lower abdomen as body turns 90 degrees to the right, and palms move upwards to finish with right at shoulder level facing away from body and left level with right armpit facing towards body.

Continue by shifting weight on to left leg, turning body back through 90 degrees, as left arm pushes forward at shoulder height, almost, palm facing body, and right fingers rest on wrist of left arm.

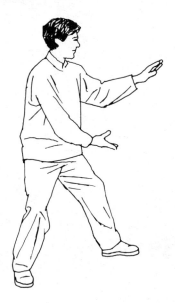

Fig. 24

Weight shifts on to right leg and left toes are raised, heel on floor, as right fingers and palm slide over top of left hand and then both palms separate at shoulder height, downward facing, elbows bent to about 90 degrees.

Weight shifts on to left leg and both palms push downward and forward steeply, then upward in a gradual ascent to shoulder height (Figure 25).

Diagonal Leaning

With weight still on left leg turn right foot through 45 degrees to face 12 on the clock, pushing both palms outwards in a slight arc as if pushing open two sliding doors, then weight shifts on to right leg and left foot turns inwards to stand parallel with right.

Weight shifts on to left foot and right foot joins it, heel raised, as right palm sweeps down and up in an arc and left sweeps across in a horizontal arc so both arms are folded across chest, left nearer the body. During these two moves you face diagonally right, then front towards 12.

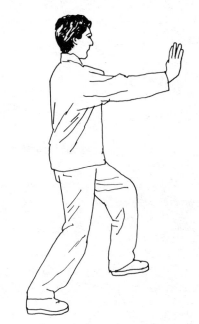

Fig. 25

Both palms form fists (Figure 26) beginning to push away from the chest, still crossed.

Weight remains on left foot as right steps out to the right towards 3/4 on the clock.

Weight shifts on to right foot, flat, and right fist moves up level with forehead as left fist descends to left hip, palm down.

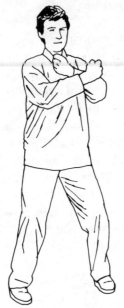

Fig. 26

following to end about six inches behind and beside left foot, heel raised; at the same time the left palm presses back and down beside left hip and right palm follows the body turn, rising open ahead of face.

Weight shifts back on to right foot as left open palm moves forward and upward, crossing above the right arm as right pulls down, to make a fist, and stops in front of the abdomen. Left heel is on the ground, toes raised; both palms are facing inwards (Figure 28).

Punch Under Elbow

Fig. 27

In this Form you move through 180 degrees by turning to your left. Weight shifts on to left foot, as you turn right open palm in a small circle in front of your face, left then right, so palm faces your nose; and left palm circles, palm flat down left then right to return to side of hip.

Weight shifts on to right foot, flat, and left heel rises so that left toes are placed opposite right heel, body turning left and both arms moving to hold a big ball, left palm up and right palm down at right side of body (Figure 27).

Body turns further left and left foot moves round to left, resting heel on ground, as right arm rises in a curve across the body to finish palm facing body, out to the right, and left palm presses down beside left hip.

Weight shifts to left foot, and trunk turns right round to 9 on the clock, right foot

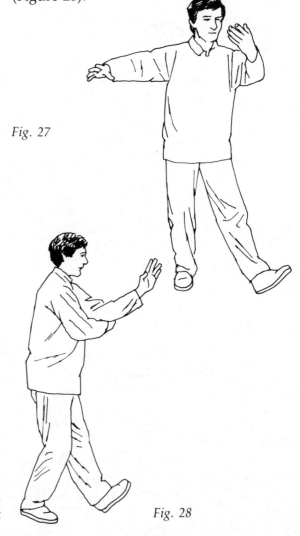

Fig. 28

Step Back and Whirl Arms (Step Back to Drive Monkey Away)

Turn body to the right and with the movement lower the right open palm in a big arc past the right outer thigh, palm up, and sweep it back and up to shoulder level so it stands out as though you were about to throw a ball with it. Simultaneously the left palm makes a small curving movement so that it is facing horizontally upwards, fingers pointing away, as if holding a saucer of milk. Left heel rises and toes only touch ground.

Step backwards with left foot, touching ground with ball of foot first then roll flat, and shift weight on to it. Rear right arm turns to present a palm down position and palm rises slightly then dips slightly to stretch out in front, 9 on clock, as left palm, upwards facing, pulls back down to left hip. Both feet are flat.

Movement repeats on left side. Step back with right foot, toes only touching ground and circle right palm to face up taking left palm back in a deep curve, palm up, then step right back with right foot, weight shifting on to it; and send left palm forward, down facing and drawing right palm, upward facing to right hip (Figure 29).

Repeat these two Forms, right and left: making four Step Back and Whirl Arms in all.

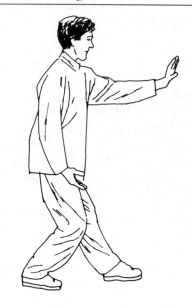

Fig. 29

Turn and Push

Place the toes of the left foot behind and slightly to side of right foot, thrusting right palm up and out a little to right, level with face; left palm descends, palm up in front of right ribs (Figure 30).

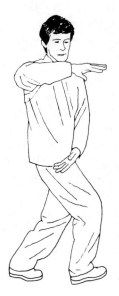

Fig. 30

Pivot left on both feet to face between 5 and 6 on the clock, bending right arm a little at elbow to face the palm down and press a little further down with the left palm.

(As you learn the Set you will appreciate that the movements flow into one another so that in the previous sentence when it says 'press a little further down with the left palm' this is really a continuation of the previous movement.)

Step a few inches towards 4 with the left foot and draw the right foot after it, heel raised, while making an arc down and across the body with the left palm to finish beside the left thigh, palm down, fingers pointing forwards; right palm pushes ahead almost vertical to finish at arm's length in front of the face (Figure 31). Drawing the back foot after the front is called Following Step.

Pivot on both feet to the right, round to 9 on the clock, ending with left foot flat and right heel raised. As you turn draw the right arm down in an arc across your left ribs and raise left arm, palm up behind and to the left of your head. This is the beginning of a repeat of the previous move, in the opposite direction and arms and legs reversed.

Step towards 11 on the clock with right foot, weight on it, and draw left in a Following Step, heel raised, as you continue your downward arc with the right palm and a push forward with the left palm. This is a repeat of the previous movement but with opposite arms and legs.

Repeat the first movement towards 7 on the clock face and the second movement towards 1. Four similar moves in all, to four different corners.

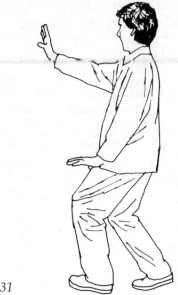

Fig. 31

Play Guitar (Lute) Right

(The original Yang-style terminology called this movement Lifting Hands, and the left-sided version (see page 49) Play Guitar. This was presumably because most people play the guitar with the left hand ahead of the right.)

Take a short step back with left foot, shifting weight on to it. As you do, turn body slightly to right and draw back left palm in front of left shoulder, raising right palm forward and upward in front of right shoulder, arm outstretched; both palms face down. Right heel raised.

Place right heel down, raising toes, with leg almost straight, bringing right palm directly in front of face, palm inward, and left palm forward opposite right elbow, palm in. (Same as previous Play Guitar but reversed.)

Brush Knee and Punch Down

Keep weight on left leg and draw right foot back to front/side of it, heel raised; palms pull back to abdomen, facing one another.

Step forward with right foot, heel down, turning body to left, raising right palm to left side of face, palm in, and left palm below right wrist, downward facing.

Shift weight to right leg, sole flat, drawing left foot, heel raised, behind/beside it; turn body to right, 9 on clock face, carrying right palm, outstretched arm, ahead of right shoulder, palm up, and left palm following it, fingertips on right forearm, lightly.

Shift weight on to left leg, raising right heel, toes remain touching ground, and take left palm down in a big arc and up back, outstretched beyond left shoulder, palm up, accompanied by a turn left of the body with right arm bending at the elbow to press down with palm close to left ribs.

Step forward to right in direction of 3 on the clock and brush the right palm across the body to finish outside the right thigh, palm down, fingers pointing ahead, while

left palm makes a fist and punches down past ear/jaw making the target of the punch the groin of an imaginary opponent – that level. As you do this Form, shift the weight on to the right leg and lean forward so that rear left leg, back and neck/head make one line (Figure 32).

White Snake Puts Out Tongue

Weight shifts on to left foot and toes of right are raised, heel on ground; right palm up, thrusting ahead and lifting level with the base of the neck; left fist rises with elbow bent oblique to, and forward of, left jaw (Figure 33).

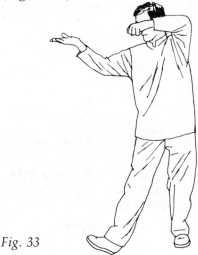

Fig. 33

Turn whole body to your left, turning the right toes in as far as you can and letting your arms travel with the body turn, up slightly past your eyes. As you make this whole body turn, through 180 degrees, shift weight on to the right foot and turn the left foot so that you face 9 on the clock. Arms continue to turn left with the body turn, the left arm finishing, palm facing up, beside the left hip, and the right palm

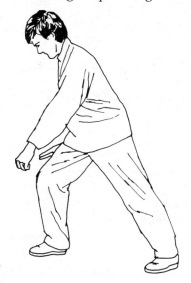

Fig. 32

thrusting forward ahead of the right shoulder, palm down, slightly raised at the wrist. Weight finally shifts back on to the left foot and the right knee moves in close taking some of the weight, tucked inside the left lower leg or calf muscle, heel raised (Figure 34).

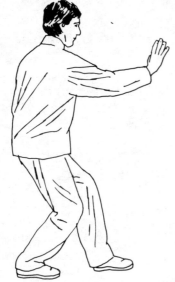

Fig. 34

Shift all the weight on to the left foot and raise right clear of ground, toes pointing down, turning body to the left and lifting left palm with open bent arm beside left shoulder, palm in, while right palm makes a small circle to move into a horizontal position.

As you turn your body back to the right, step forward with the right foot, sole flat, toes turned out a little and push forward with left palm, vertical, as you draw right palm, upward facing, back to your right hip, raising left heel from ground, toes touching.

Pat Foot to Tame Tiger

(This is a long Form to describe so as you follow it simply treat it as several Forms in terms of how you absorb it, to avoid a sense of over complication.)

Bring the left foot forward resting heel only on the ground, taking the right palm backward and upward in a big arc to finish just behind the right ear; left palm pulls back ahead of left hip, downward facing, arm almost straight.

Weight shifts on to the left foot and right foot makes a head-high toe-kick, straight ahead; right hand sweeps forward, palm down, to slap the ankle/foot of the right leg and left palm sweeps backward and upward in a big arc, ending just behind head, palm out, elbow slightly bent (Figure 35).

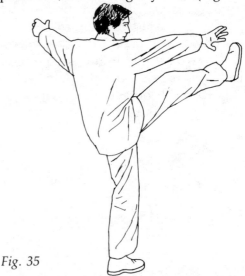

Fig. 35

Bring the right foot back down beside left, but on the *outside* of it and as soon as it rests flat on the ground you lift the left foot – a quick exchange; right palm pulls back fractionally, vertical, facing away from face and left palm comes forward in front of chest, downward facing (Figure 36).

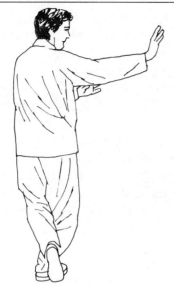

Fig. 36

Swivel towards 6 on the clock and step towards 4/5 with the left foot, bringing both arms down, fists clenched, past the abdomen, left finishing shoulder height towards your left front corner and right in front of your abdomen, palms face down. Weight mainly on left foot.

Trunk turns to the right, and head looks right, left elbow bending to bring the fist close to the forehead and right fist rising to left upper chest (Figure 37).

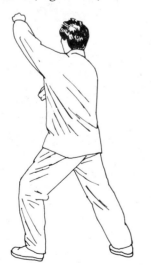

Fig. 37

Weight shifts on to the right leg and left foot turns in, right, as you bring your left palm, upward facing, in front of your chest, and right palm, downward facing, pushes across your left forearm.

Weight shifts on to left foot and right palm thrusts out ahead of right shoulder, palm down and bent slightly upwards while left palm pulls back to left hip, upward facing.

Bring the right foot in an arc to the left instep and then step towards 3 on the clock, putting weight on to it. Left palm travels down, back, up and forward in an arc to finish high, just above head and in front of it, while right palm makes an arc back to the right hip, palm up.

Kick forward, upward to head height with left foot, slapping ankle/foot with left downward palm and swinging right palm back, up and out to side, head height, palm outward facing. As before but reversed.

Bring left foot down beside right but on *outside* of it and as before immediately lift right foot; left palm making a small arc to face almost down and right palm coming forward in front of chest, almost downward facing.

Turn body right towards 1/2 on the clock and step in same direction with right foot, shifting weight on to it. As before swing both palms, in fist formation, low past the abdomen so that right fist ends obliquely forward on right side of shoulder and left below it, to left of right elbow, palms downward facing.

Finish by bringing right fist close to right side of the forehead and left fist to upper part of right chest, turning head to look left.

Turn Left and Strike

Weight shifts on to left leg as body turns to left, right toes rise and foot begins to turn in, fists opening and drawing closer to front of chest, where they cross, right palm up and left down.

Left palm continues to cross right forearm and as body turns further left it pushes out to left side, level with left shoulder, and right palm descends in front of right hip (Figure 38); weight shifts on to right foot, now pointing ahead.

Bring left foot close to right as you turn body slightly left then right, bringing left palm down into a fist in front of abdomen and circling right arm in a big curve, back, up, over and down to rest palm on left forearm.

Step towards 7/8 on the clock with left foot and shift weight on to it, as you strike up and forward with left fist, palm facing body; right palm follows attached to left forearm.

Threading Palm and Crouch Down

Toes of left foot rise as weight shifts to right leg, and left open palm draws back and out to side of left shoulder and right palm thrusts forward; trunk turns left.

As weight shifts to left leg step forward with right leg beside it bringing right palm across in front of the face, fist clenched and left palm down and across in front of abdomen, also in a fist. Palms close into fists gradually and end with fists facing body (Figure 39).

Slowly squat down on the left leg and slide the right foot towards 10 on the clock until it is almost straight. (Take care with this movement; to begin with squat down only a few inches and be aware of your lower back, sacral region; do *not* force this posture.) At the same time the right arm descends and the left fist threads across it, outside it, and upwards.

Push right fist out along line of right leg as body turns a little right and draw left fist up higher behind left side of head (Figure 40).

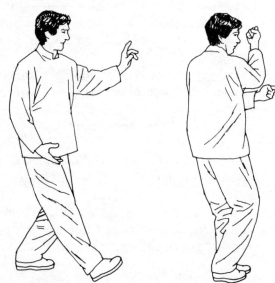

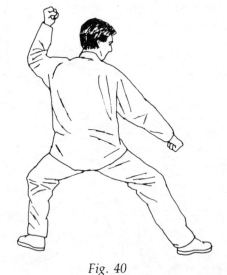

Fig. 38   *Fig. 39*   *Fig. 40*

Ward Off Standing On One Leg

(Begin this next Form with care to avoid any excess strain on the right knee.) Shift weight on to right leg, turning toes out and lift the right fist as you lower the left fist so that they are both level with one another; both fists continue to have palms facing same direction as before.

Shift weight completely on to right leg and raise left heel as you circle the open right palm inward and back to 'point' forward again, palm down; left fist opens, presses down to waist level and moves forward close to right elbow, twisting inwards (Figure 41).

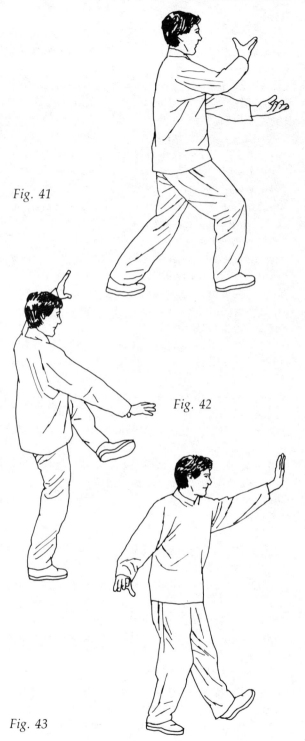

Fig. 41

Continue by raising left knee so thigh is horizontal but lower leg turns inward a little so that sole of foot turns to angle of 45 degrees to ground, raising the left palm, facing away from body, in front of forehead and lowering right palm, facing inside of left calf muscle (Figure 42).

Fig. 42

Step forward with the left foot, heel down first, turning body to the left and pushing higher with left palm and drawing right palm towards right hip. (Remember that the body moves *as a whole* and arm movements in particular can be seen as results, in a sense, of body/leg movements, rather than as independent, isolated actions.) (Figure 43.)

Shift weight on to left leg, flat sole, and raise right heel, lowering left palm ahead of left shoulder and pushing right palm a little forward as body turns front again.

Raise right knee, horizontal thigh, bringing right palm up and back *above* the head, palm upwards facing and fingers pointing across to left, while left palm lowers to inside of right knee.

Fig. 43

Right Single Whip

Lower right foot and step backwards with it, keeping most weight still on left leg, bringing right palm out to the right, forward and down in an arc to the front, raising left palm to shoulder level (Figure 44).

Weight shifts back on to right leg, body turns right; keep left sole flat and lower both hands to hip level.

Bend left elbow to raise palm up and in, inward facing in front of chest, and raise right palm to rest on left wrist.

Weight shifts back to left leg, body turning towards 9 on clock, and both palms press forwards to 9, vertical, facing face.

As weight shifts on to right leg, raise left toes and circle left palm to left and bend wrist back.

Shift weight on to left foot, body turning right and left toes turning right at same time; raise right heel and bend left wrist down so that fingers and thumb meet to form a hook or beak and send left arm out just rising above horizontal to your left.

Step towards 3 on the clock face with right foot, shifting weight on to it, and push out ahead of face with right palm (Figure 45).

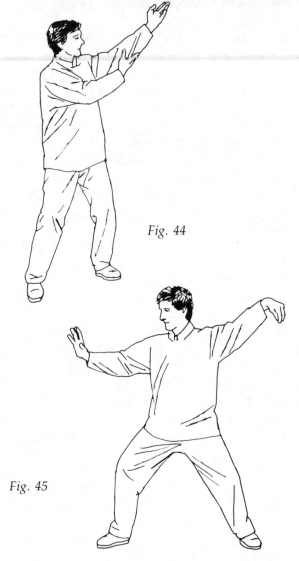

Fig. 44

Fig. 45

Wave Hands Like Clouds

(In this Form you move along a straight line to the right, trunk turning right and left.)

Shift weight to the left leg and lower right palm down then up facing body, opposite left armpit.

Open left hook/beak palm to face away from body, palm vertical and draw right palm slightly up and across body to right, turning trunk a little to the left.

Shift weight on to right leg, right arm continuing to arc to above right shoulder, arm bent at elbow and palm facing body, as left palm lowers in front of abdomen, palm facing body (Figure 46).

(Though feet move closer together and then apart they remain parallel to one another pointing towards 12 on the clock.)

Bring left foot closer to right, below left

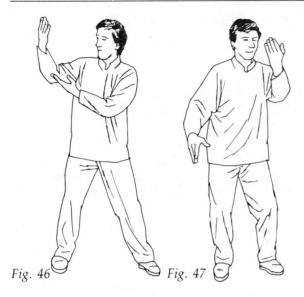

Fig. 46   *Fig. 47*

hip joint, pushing right hand out to the right, palm turning away from body and left palm rising to right armpit, facing body. Turn head to look right (Figure 47).

Shift weight on to left leg as your body and head turn 180 degrees left to look left, bringing left palm up past face and out to left side of face and taking right palm, inward facing, in a big arc down across lower abdomen and up towards left armpit.

Step out to right with right leg and push palms further left, facing left, accompanied by trunk left turn.

Weight shifts to right leg as left arm descends and right arm rises to push out right once more. Then bring left foot close to right again and repeat the same movements to push out left with palms. Step right again finishing the leftward push, then shift weight on to right foot.

To complete this Form, push once more out to the right and bring the left foot to the right foot again.

(In this Form there are five pushes: right, left, right, left, right.)

Part Wild Horse Mane

As weight shifts on to the left leg, both palms pull in to the right side of the body as if holding a ball – left palm level with left shoulder and right palm level with left hip.

Step out right with right foot towards 3 on clock face and shift weight on to it, flat sole, raising right palm, upward facing, level with right shoulder and lowering left palm, downward facing, level with left hip (Figure 48).

Shift weight on to left leg and raise right toes, turning right foot about 45 degrees to right, turning body with it, and holding a big ball in front of body as you step up with the left foot, heel raised, and shift weight on to flat right foot, and turn body back towards 3.

Step forward with left foot towards 3 and flat sole as weight shifts on to it. Raise left palm and lower right palm as in previous Form. (The Form is the same, done on the left side.)

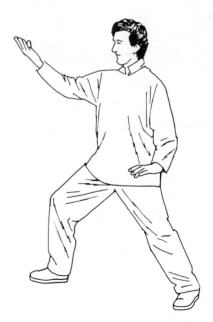

Fig. 48

High Pat On Horse

Draw the right foot up just to the side of, and behind, the left – left heel raised, and turn left palm into an upward facing position with a gentle circular action, raising right palm to face down, beside right shoulder (Figure 49).

Shift weight on to right foot, lowering heel, and take a small step forward with left foot, turning trunk first right then left as you do so; bring left palm down, facing up, to side of left thigh, and push forward with right palm ahead of right shoulder, palm down sloping at an angle of about 45 degrees to the vertical (Figure 50).

(Note: the angles of foot, trunk, palm, and so forth are all approximate and will vary with the build of the student, preferences of the teacher and so on.)

Kick With Right Heel

Raise the left heel and bring right palm back to right shoulder as you push left palm downward facing ahead and turn body a little to left.

Step with left heel towards 1/2 on the clock and bring right palm forward turning left palm to face it.

Weight shifts on to left leg as right palm moves up and down, palm outward facing, to the right, level with shoulder, and left palm moves down and up to the left, level with left shoulder, outward facing (Figure 51).

Bring right foot close to left, heel raised, and cross both arms in front of chest, palms facing body.

Raise right knee, leg bent, then straighten leg to kick horizontally forward with right heel, sending both palms out to the sides.

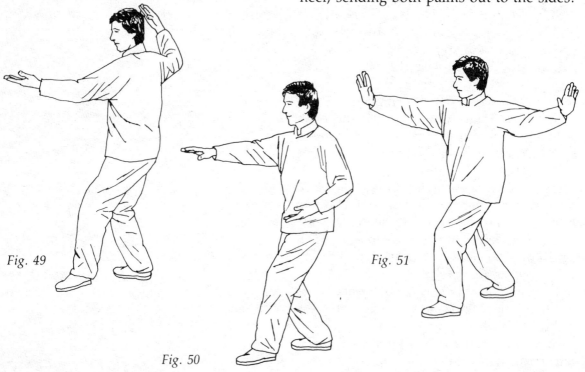

Fig. 49

Fig. 51

Fig. 50

Strike With Both Fists

Lower right leg, thigh horizontal, and bring both palms down alongside right thigh, upward facing.

Step down with right foot towards 5 on clock and lower both palms level with hips.

Form fists with both palms as you shift weight on to the right foot, bringing both fists up, out and round as though to strike someone on the ears simultaneously with both fists, using the thumb edges and first knuckles (Figure 52).

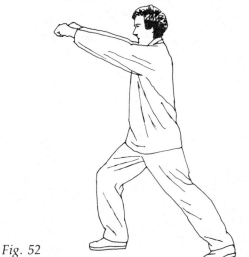

Fig. 52

Kick With Left Heel

Weight shifts on to left leg and right toes rise as palms push up and down in a slight curve to the sides of the body, turning body towards 3 on clock.

Shift weight back to right leg drawing left foot close to it, heel raised, and bring both palms, inward facing in front of body, left palm just ahead of right, arms slightly bent.

Raise left thigh parallel to ground and kick upward with left heel, pushing arms out to the sides, palms facing outward.

Punch With Concealed Fist

Lower left foot beside right, toes only touching ground, and bring both palms in front of face, left open and right making a fist (Figure 53).

Step towards 1/2 on the clock with the left foot and turn body to the right as you lower both fists level with the right hip, both palms up and right fist resting in palm of left hand.

Weight shifts on to left leg as right fist punches forward to abdomen level and left palm draws back to left hip, making a fist, palm up.

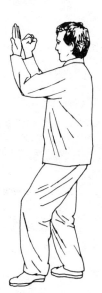

Fig. 53

Needle At Sea Bottom

Weight stays on left leg as right foot makes a half pace towards left foot, heel raised, right palm open, inward facing, coming back in front of right thigh and left palm, open, downward facing, pushes forward in front of chest.

Weight shifts on to right leg and left heel is raised as right palm curves back, up and forward in front of right shoulder and left palm curves out and down above left knee, body turning with the palms to the right.

Slide left toes a few inches forward and turn body to front again, drawing left palm to side of left hip joint and thrusting right palm down in a 45 degree angle to vertical, leaning trunk a little forward from hips (Figure 54).

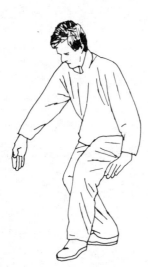

Fig. 54

Fan Penetrates Back (Flash the Arm)

Raise left foot just below right knee level and bring right hand back closer to the body, pushing left palm forward and across to face in, just back from right wrist.

Take a deep step forward with left foot and push left arm straight ahead, palm in and bent up at the wrist, drawing right palm, outward facing, to the side of the right temple and forehead (Figure 55).

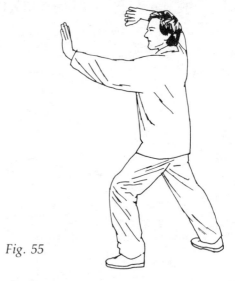

Fig. 55

Kick With Right and Left Feet

Turn the right foot, while it is still bearing little weight, round to 6 on the clock, and shift weight on to it, turning the trunk in the same direction and in the same movement turning the left foot in the same direction: right turns out, left turns in. As you do so push both palms out to the side, facing away from the body. Look right. Weight is mainly on the right foot.

Weight shifts on to left leg and at same time turns left toes a little to the right, drawing right foot close to left, heel raised;

turning trunk to the right bring both palms down in arcs, across the body and up to cross in front of the chest, facing in, right furthest from body.

Turn both palms away from the body and push right palm straight ahead, almost straight arm, and push left palm out to the side, shoulder height, as you lift right thigh and kick upwards with toe (Figure 56).

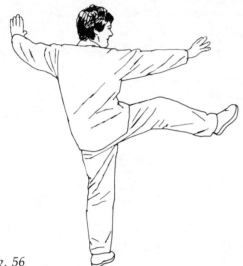

Fig. 56

Lower the right foot by bending the knee then stepping out towards 10 on the clock, heel only touching, and draw right palm back a little, turning palm in, as left palm pushes down past left hip and up to face inside of right forearm. Shift weight on to right flat foot and push left palm out towards 9 on the clock sending right palm back and to the side, palm out, shoulder level, looking towards 9.

Left foot comes forward beside right, heel raised, arms cross as before but left furthest from body, then separate the arms and kick up with left toe as before.

Brush Left and Right Knees

Lower the left leg by bending the knee and place foot close to right, heel raised; right arm bending, and palm coming in to face the eyes as head turns towards it, left palm drawing back towards and down the body to rest, downward facing, at waist level.

Step towards 9 with the left foot and shift weight on to it, bringing left palm forward and across the body to 'brush' above left knee and stop on outside of thigh, fingers pointing front, while right palm pushes forward at chin level towards 9, body and head turning in same direction.

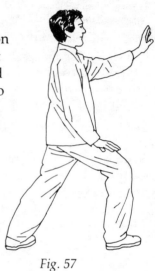

Fig. 57

Weight shifts back on to right foot and left toes rise and turn a little to the left, as left palm makes a little scooping action, face upwards, and right arm begins to bend at the elbow bringing right palm back towards the face.

Raise the left palm and turn head to look at it as you shift weight on to left flat foot, right foot coming close to and slightly ahead of left, heel raised. Whole body follows the head turn left, and right palm, facing down, lowers to level with waist.

Step straight towards 9 with the right foot, 'brush' the right knee and push forward as before, this time with left palm (Figure 57).

Step Up and Punch

Weight shifts back on to left foot and right toes are raised as left palm draws back a little closer to the body, palm up, and right palm pushes across left forearm, palm down.

Right toes turn a little to the right and weight shifts on to right foot as right palm pushes diagonally forward right, facing away, and left palm curves right and then left in front of waist.

Step forward on to left heel, pushing left palm up and forward left, slowly making a fist, palm inward facing, and drawing right palm back to right hip, palm up, also making a fist.

Weight shifts on to left flat foot and right fist, inward facing, punches forward and up in front of face while left fist comes back, turning in a little, palm down, resting under the right wrist (Figure 58).

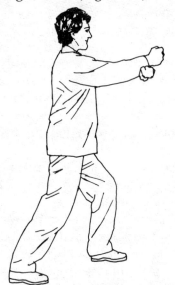

Fig. 58

As if Closing a Door

Step forward with right foot, heel raised, just behind and to side of left, and open both palms, turning them upwards and slightly bent upwards at the wrists (Figure 59).

Take a short step forward with left foot as you shift weight on to right, and draw palms back towards body, inward facing, then stretch out left leg to touch ground with heel, and push down with both palms towards abdomen, and then forward, palms facing away from body, as you shift weight fully on to flat left foot.

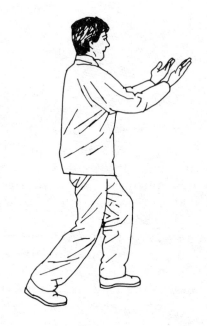

Fig. 59

Wave Hands Like Clouds

This is a repeat of the earlier move, moving left instead of right.

Turn right foot a little to the right and trunk with it, slowly shifting weight on to right leg, and turning left toes in to run parallel with right foot; right arm curves slightly up and down, away to the right, palm facing away from body, and left palm drops to the right, scooping up to lie at waist height almost below right elbow.

Bring weight slowly on to left foot, and draw left palm up across chest to stand to the left of the head, palm facing face as you look at it, and right arm coming down across abdomen and scooping up almost below left elbow.

Bring right foot closer to left, turn left palm away from face, and straighten left elbow a little and begin to bring right palm back towards its previous position.

Take both palms back across to the first position, turning trunk and head as before and shift weight on to right leg.

Step left with no weight on left foot and begin to bring arms back to second position as before.

Shift weight on to left leg and complete the movement to the left; then repeat the whole movement turning to the right again; then complete it once more to the left.

Turn Right and Strike

Step diagonally backwards towards 5 with the left leg and bend the right with weight on it, lowering and turning the left palm up in front of the waist and pushing the right palm, downward facing, across the left forearm and out at chin height towards 10.

Weight shifts back on to left leg; raise right heel, turning the trunk to the left and looking towards 9. Bring right palm back in a fist, palm facing body, in front of the waist, and left palm moves down, back, up and down once more in a circle to finish behind the right forearm, palm down.

Step towards 10 with the right foot and punch upward and forward in same direction with right fist (an uppercut), while left palm follows the right forearm without losing position (Figure 60).

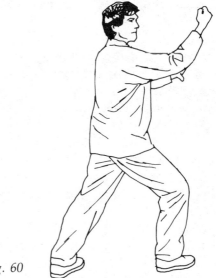

Fig. 60

Fair Lady Works With Shuttles

Weight shifts on to left leg; raise right toes and open right fist into a palm inward facing; then shift weight on to right foot, flat, trunk turning to face 10 on the clock, left palm pushing out in front of body at shoulder height and right palm going down and up to cover left inner elbow.

Bring left foot close up beside right, toes only touching, drawing left palm, oblique to the ground, in front of abdomen, and right palm, upward facing, to the right hip (Figure 61).

Step towards 7 with left foot, flat, and shift weight on to it, while turning left forearm so that palm faces towards body, at neck height, and right palm fingers rest near the wrist of the left arm (Figure 62).

Draw right foot up behind and to the side of the left, toes touching, and move both arms to the left, lowering the left elbow.

Settle weight back on to right foot, flat, and step forward a few inches on to left toes, turning body right, and bringing right palm, inward facing, to the right lower ribs, and bringing left palm round at head height, palm inward facing.

Step towards 7 with left foot, flat, and turn body towards 9, pushing straight ahead with right vertical palm and pulling left palm, facing 9, just above forehead (Figure 63).

Weight shifts on to right leg, and left toes lift to leave heel on ground, drawing left palm forward and in front of chest, slightly bent, and pushing; right palm pulls back to push across top of left forearm, palm facing left forearm.

Shift weight on to left foot, flat, bringing left palm down, upward facing, in front of left lower ribs, and turning right palm,

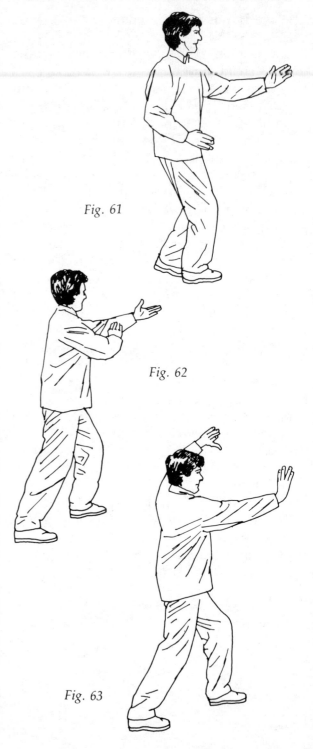

Fig. 61

Fig. 62

Fig. 63

facing out, at shoulder height, to right front side of body; body turns right with it (Figure 64).

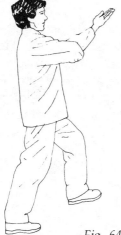

Fig. 64

Weight stays on left foot as right foot, toes touching, comes up close to left instep, and left palm draws back to left hip, and right palm draws back to press down in front of abdomen.

Step towards 10 with right foot, flat, (this is same movement done on the other side), and push right arm ahead of right shoulder turning palm almost flat, while left palm fingers rest on inside of right wrist, and shift weight on to right foot.

Bring left foot close to right instep, toes touching, and draw both arms towards right rear, turning body right and lowering right elbow.

Settle weight back on to left foot, raising right heel, and turn right palm upwards near right temple while left palm pushes up in front of face.

Step towards 10 with right foot, flat, and shift weight on to it, turning body right further and finishing with right palm just above forehead and left palm pushing further ahead of the face, palm facing away from face.

Step Back With Cross-over Palm

Weight shifts on to left leg and right toes lift, heel on ground. Bring left palm down in an arc to the left hip, palm down, and right arm goes forward at shoulder level, palm inward facing, arm almost straight.

Step back with right foot and keep weight on left foot as you push the right palm forward and upward, upward facing, ahead of the face and bring the right arm down and across in a fist to rest under the left elbow.

Press Down Palms With Empty Step

Weight shifts on to right leg and left foot turns in to bring body facing towards 2 on the clock as the right palm is drawn back in front of the lower chest and the left palm comes up to face the left side of the temple/forehead.

Weight shifts on to right leg as right foot turns in and left foot turns out, heel raised; simultaneously the left palm descends to just above the right knee, palm down, fingers pointing across, and right palm pulls back towards right hip. Facing 3 on the clock (Figure 65).

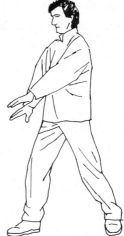

Fig. 65

Stand On One Leg Holding Out Palm

Raise the right knee, thigh parallel to ground, lower leg straight down with toes pointing down as left palm draws back to the side of the left chest level with shoulder and right palm extends ahead of body, palm upward facing; body turning a little to the left (Figure 66).

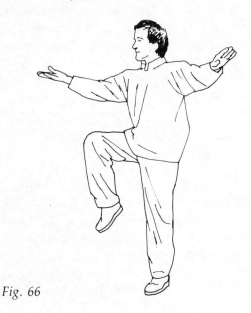

Fig. 66

turns upward facing, going back, down and up in an arc beyond the right shoulder with the left palm making a fist and descending level with the waist, palm down.

Step towards 2 with left foot, shifting half of weight on to it in the Horse Riding Stance (Figure 67) and turn trunk towards 3. Left fist is pushed down and forward above left knee by the right palm which comes down and rests, palm down, on the left forearm.

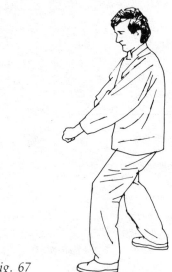

Fig. 67

Push Forearm With Horse Stance

Weight follows right leg as you step down towards 5 with that leg, foot flat, turning body to the right and raising the left heel, toes touching. The right palm turns to face down and draws back just ahead of right hip as left palm extends ahead of left shoulder, palm in a vertical plane facing inwards.

Weight remains on right leg as left foot is brought up beside it, toes only touching, and torso turns far round to the right so that eyes can look back at right palm which

Turn Body With Large Strokes

Weight shifts on to right leg, raising left toes, and both palms open, and turn to face right with right body turn.

Turn left foot towards 2, lowering sole flat on ground, and shift weight on to it, as left palm rises, arm almost completely bent, palm twisting out to face left; right arm extends almost straight, ahead of right shoulder, palm up. Then bring right foot up to left, as if feet are standing to attention and raise right palm a couple of inches higher (Figures 68 and 69).

Turn body about 90 degrees right, using right foot to pivot, then sit down on right foot with left foot, heel raised, resting slightly ahead of right; right palm rises, facing inwards, ahead of right temple, arm half bent, and left arm straightens a little, but still bent, so that left palm faces diagonally downwards and inwards ahead of left shoulder.

Left foot steps backwards leaving weight on right leg, and right palm moves away from the body towards 11, palm up and turned inward, with left palm descending just behind right elbow, palm down (Figure 70).

Turn left toes to the left and shift weight on to left leg turning right foot inwards to the left using the ball of the foot as a pivot; turn trunk right round to the left in line with left foot and bring left palm, slowly making a fist, round to the left hip, palm facing upward; note that left elbow is held a few inches away from the body so that forearm/fist is pointing inwards. At the same time the right palm slowly makes a fist, and, synchronizing with the body turn, travels past the face, descends in an arc beyond the left ribs and back across the body to the right side, arm bent at the elbow so that the fist is held at solar plexus height, palm up (Figure 71: 72 reverse view).

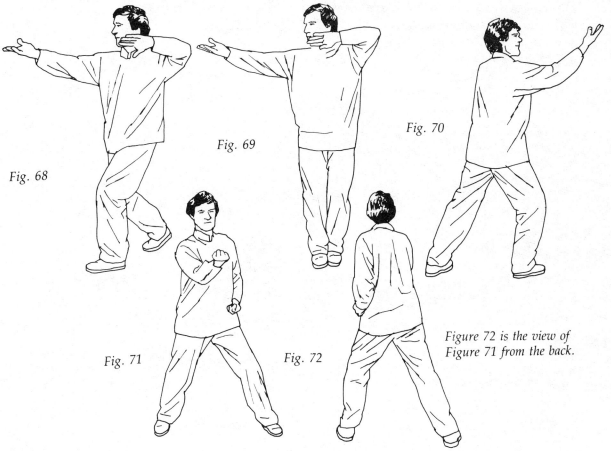

Fig. 68

Fig. 69

Fig. 70

Fig. 71

Fig. 72

Figure 72 is the view of Figure 71 from the back.

Swinging Palms and Crouching Step (Single Whip Squatting Down)

Shift weight on to right leg turning trunk a little to the right and raising the right fist level with the forehead, palm down, as left fist pushes down and back below and behind left hip (Figure 73).

Left foot turns towards 5 on clock and weight shifts on to left leg as both palms open, left rising to solar plexus level, palm facing body, elbow bent, and right palm is lowered to outside of right thigh, gradually turning to face inwards (left).

Bring right foot, toes only touching, beside left foot, continuing with right palm movement inwards to finish in front of lower abdomen, palm obliquely downwards, and left palm coming in and across body to rest fingers on lower right forearm.

Weight moves on to right leg and torso turns to the right (Figure 74) as the left knee is raised, thigh parallel to ground and lower leg vertical; both arms move right, left fingers still 'attached' to right forearm, as right arm opens and extends to the right to form a hook/beak.

Extend the left leg towards 2 to place left foot flat on ground (Figure 75) and bend right leg into a crouching, squatting or sitting down position (exercising caution over depth of knee bend to avoid excessive strain at the knee and sacral region) and then lowering left palm, inward facing, down past the right chest, abdomen, groin and extending it along the inside of the left leg, palm facing inwards (Figure 76).

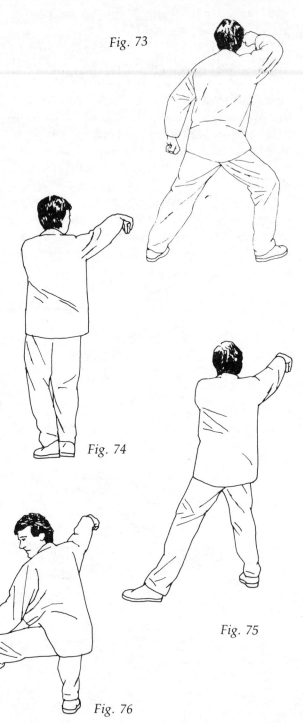

Fig. 73

Fig. 74

Fig. 75

Fig. 76

Step Up and Cross Fists

(This move comes from the Yang-style move called Step Up To Form The Seven Stars, but here the position of the right foot has been changed.)

Rise up (carefully) to put weight on to left leg and push left palm up and forward, arm almost extended, facing inward, and draw right palm forward down and back behind right hip, in an arc, fingers still in hook/beak position, palm facing backwards (Figure 77).

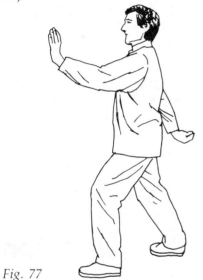

Fig. 77

Bring right foot forward to rest on ball of foot ahead of left foot, at the same time making the left palm into a fist and bringing the right palm forward and upward in a fist so that both fists cross at the wrists in front of the chest, arms slightly bent, left fist on top and palms down.

Stand On One Leg To Ride The Tiger

Bringing the right foot back one step, shift the weight on to it and bring the left open palm across the front at chin height, palm inwards facing, vertical, drawing right open palm, downwards facing, back to the right hip.

Shift body weight firmly on to right leg as body turns to face 3 and left foot slides a little closer to the right, heel raised, as the left palm draws back to left hip, facing down, and right palm makes a big arc, up, across and down body from right to left, to finish, palm up, above left thigh (Figure 78).

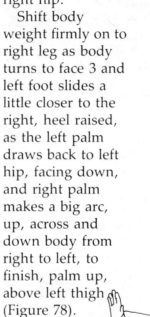

Fig. 78

Raise left foot, toes pointing a little inwards, as right palm pushes upward and forward in front of right shoulder and left palm goes back, down, up and sideways in a hook/beak (Figure 79).

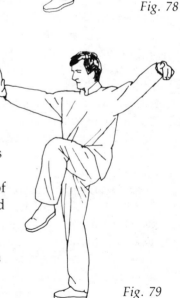

Fig. 79

Sweep Lotus With Leg

Combine the descending weight of the left leg, the rotation of the arms and shoulders to the right, and the turning of the trunk to the right, to bring the left foot across to step to the right of the right foot. The extended left palm, inward facing, helps this action as the right palm pulls down to the right hip, upward facing. Trunk is now facing 5 on clock (Figure 80). (This movement may be difficult at first; if so, compromise by turning less far to the right until your joints and balance improve.)

Turn further right on the balls of both feet, round to 9, thrusting the left palm, inward facing, diagonally downward and upward in front of the face, and 'cupping' the left elbow with the open right palm – not touching (Figure 81).

Without pausing, the body continues to turn right on the balls of both feet so that you face 12 on the clock and the right palm rises past and close to the face to push out right towards 3, followed by the left palm which presses down, inward facing, in front of the right ribs (Figure 82).

(The next movement is difficult to describe clearly but with experiment you will grasp it.) The trunk turns a little to the right and back again left to face 12. This small torso twist is brought about by raising the right foot to the left and up in an arc so that it swings back to the right at about shoulder level (or lower depending on flexibility). At the same time, both palms swing in unison from right to left, in turn slapping the passing foot, sharply (Figure 83).

(To begin with, raise the right foot only about twelve to eighteen inches and make small, token movements with the hands, so that you get the notion of what is involved.)

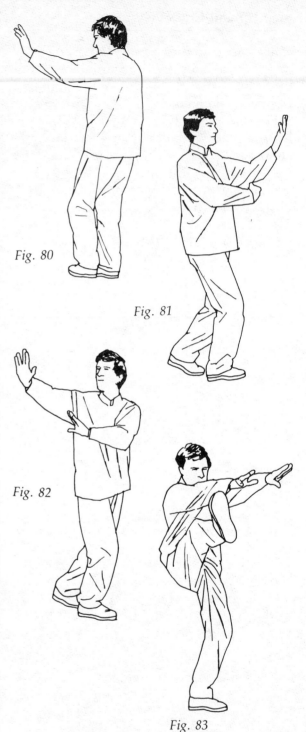

Fig. 80

Fig. 81

Fig. 82

Fig. 83

Bend The Bow To Shoot The Tiger

As you complete the swing with the arms in the previous Form, you lower the right leg to the position shown in Figure 84 so that the thigh is horizontal, lower leg vertical, and turn the trunk towards 2 on the clock, pushing the left palm out to your right at shoulder height and pressing down with the right palm just in front of the right ribs, palm obliquely down.

Slowly lower both palms, downward facing, and bring them across the body at waist height as you lower the right leg towards 4, only the heel resting on the ground.

Flatten the right foot and shift weight on to it, toes pointing to 4, and turn the torso in the same direction, bringing both palms, slowly forming fists, in a downward and upward arc to the right side of the body. Both fists are almost at the same height, right slightly higher, palms down. Imagine you are grasping the ends of a small bow. Look right towards the right fist (Figure 85).

Turn the trunk towards 3 and twist both fists inward and outward as if bending the bow, sending the right fist a little further out to the right and upward and the left fist out to the left and forward. Look front (Figure 86).

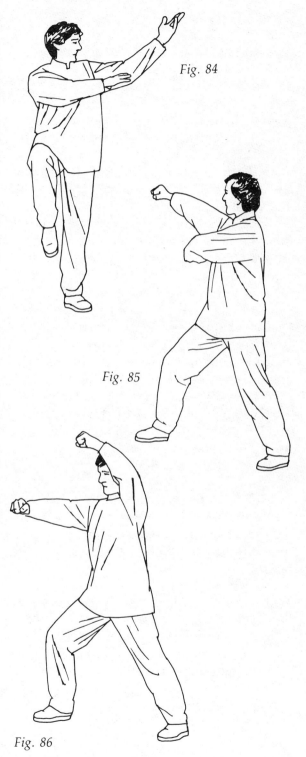

Fig. 84

Fig. 85

Fig. 86

Strike, Parry and Punch

Weight shifts back on to left leg and right toes rise as the left fist opens into a palm, facing body diagonally upward, with right fist opening at the same time, palm approaching and facing left elbow.

Lower right toes to the ground, turning them inward as you do so, and draw left palm back to left hip, pushing right palm away at shoulder height and turning trunk to the left.

Bring right foot, heel raised, close to left foot, bringing right palm back and down in an arc, fist clenched, palm down, in front of abdomen, while left palm rises, palm down, in front of the chest and body turns back to the right.

Right foot steps forward on to the heel, toes out, as right fist rises and strikes forward in front of the chest, palm up, and left palm presses down in front of left hip.

Weight shifts on to the right leg and torso turns right. Left foot steps forward on to the left heel as the left palm pushes forward in front of the left shoulder and right fist draws back to the right hip, palm facing upward.

Weight shifts on to the left foot, flat, and the right fist punches forward to shoulder height as the left open palm returns to touch the inside of the right forearm. Look ahead.

Ward Off, Roll Back, Press and Push Right

This sequence is a repetition of the Form done early in the Set, except that it is done on the right instead of the left. As an interesting exercise, see if you can work it out for yourself, referring to the instructions on page 52.

Crossing Hands

Weight shifts on to the left foot, and body turns to face 12, as you move from the push position in the previous Form. Left toes turn right as the weight changes. At the same time turn the right toes to the left as the weight changes (Figure 87). The left palm follows the leftward turn of the body and the right palm remains extended to the right from the previous Form.

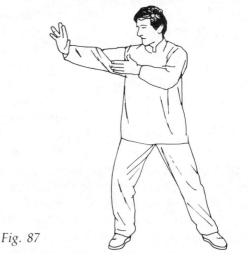

Fig. 87

Shift weight a little on to the right foot and turn the left toes further right to point towards 10 then lower the weight on to the left leg, straightening the right leg and pushing the left palm further left, looking at the left hand (Figure 88).

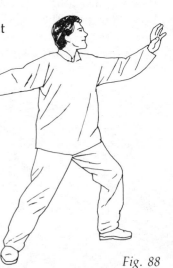

Fig. 88

Weight shifts on to the right leg and the left toes turn inwards so that both feet are parallel facing 12. Bring both palms down across the body and cross them in front of the chest, facing inwards, elbows down a little, so that the cross is made to the right side of the chest. Right arm closer to the body.

Bring the left foot in to the right, feet hip width apart, and bring the cross to the centre of the chest.

Closing

Turn both palms to face downward and draw them apart. When they reach the armpits turn the fingers to face the front. As the palms press down, straighten the legs – palms downward moving, body upward moving – and bring the palms to the sides of the thighs, fingers pointing down.

Left foot joins the right foot. This is the end of the Set.

Legs And Feet Exercises

If you become interested in and appreciative of Tai Chi, you will join the ranks of those people who can find pleasure in little things. You will see the importance and value of little things, and understand that they make all the difference. This echoes the old English proverb-poem:

For the want of a nail a horse shoe was lost
For the want of a horse shoe a horse was lost
For the want of a horse a rider was lost
For the want of a rider a message was lost
For the want of a message a battle was lost
For the want of a battle a kingdom was lost
And all for the want of a nail . . .

If you bear this old proverb in mind it will help you to become interested in your feet. Everything else is above the feet; they are the mobile foundations of your body. One Chinese belief places a man or woman's head as the equivalent of Heaven, the hands the equivalent of Earth, and the feet as the equivalent of Man. Though Heaven is higher it depends on Earth. Though Earth is higher is depends on Man.

Observe your own naked foot and note that the inside edge, the instep, is an arch. The inside edge of the foot, the arch, is designed to be raised. It follows from this that any tendency for the ankle joint to bend inwards is contrary to the design of the foot.

1. Stand upright as you usually do and notice whether your ankle joints have a tendency to fall inwards. This is the case with many people. If they do, push your weight more towards the outside edges of your feet – release – push out – release. Keep your knees slightly bent. Except as an intentional exercise, never lock your knees back because it throws out the alignment of your spine. If you become tired, sit down, but do not follow any inclination to lock the knees to 'rest'.

2. Imagine that you are standing on railway lines. The lines are the same width apart as the distance between your hips. Imagine also that there is a pencil line drawn from the middle of your heel, along the middle of your foot, ending in the middle of the spread of your toes. Put your heel down in front of you to make a step, as though you were aiming to place the start of the pencil line down exactly in the middle of the right-hand railway line. Bend your toes upwards as you place your heel down, then as you settle the sole of the foot on to the ground, you 'roll' your foot out, as though it were a piece of rolled up carpet, so that your foot is completely flat. Your shin bone is vertical above your foot and your ankle bone is straight. Step forward with the other foot in the same way and continue to the limit of your space, turn round and go back.

   At first you may have to bend forward to look at your feet to see what is going on, but with training you will be able to sense what is going on with the feet and legs and stand upright. If your ankles habitually fall inwards this new use of the feet will feel strange and you will notice new muscular actions in the lower leg. An interesting thing to do is to examine the soles of your shoes; where they are more worn away are obviously the areas which come in for most weight bearing and this can also tell you something about your usual way of walking and standing.

   As you walk forwards in the above fashion, vary the angle of your foot. Sometimes turn your toes out, and at other times keep them straight in line with your heels. If you are still not sure about the exercise, try it without your shoes on. Do not overly tense your feet to produce the rolling down carpet action. Find just what force is needed.

3. Still stand on the railway lines. Take one pace forward and bend your front knee. Keep your rear leg extended but slightly bent at the knee. The front toes point forward and the rear foot is turned out about 45 degrees. This is an approximation of the most widely used stance or leg position in Tai Chi. It is called the Bow stance or sometimes the Bow and Arrow stance. The front leg is bent like a bow and the rear leg is stretched like the bow string. But not taut. It is an approximation because there are a number of finer points which need to be followed before it becomes accurate. Keep your shin bone in the front leg in line with your foot; that is, the ankle joint is in the vertical plane. The front knee does not extend beyond the front toes. The thigh bone of the rear leg is of course at an angle to the pelvis, at the thigh joint, and the pelvis is as near vertical as anatomy permits. You have a feeling of partially 'sitting down' on the rear leg. Your trunk is upright.

Try slowly shifting your weight back and forth from rear leg to front leg. When your weight is more centred over the rear leg this is called the Back stance or Rear stance, and this too is a common position in Tai Chi.

Now, shift your weight once more from Bow to Rear stance and as you go into Rear stance raise the toes of the front foot so that only the heel rests on the ground. With your feet in this position, try turning the toes of the foot inwards or outwards some 45 degrees and put the sole of the foot on the ground. These few manoeuvres are used a lot in Tai Chi and to practise them in advance will prepare you well for moving about in the Forms.

4. Take the Rear stance again with the right foot in front, toes raised. Turn the toes in 45 degrees and put the foot down flat. Now, shift your weight on to that foot, turn your pelvis a little and put most of your weight on the turned in foot. This is the Turned In stance. Still in the Turned In stance, lift the heel of the non-weight-bearing foot, the left, so that only the ball of the foot is on the ground. Turn that foot on its ball, to the left, then step diagonally left with it, so that it points in the opposite direction to the one you were in when you began this manoeuvre. Shift your weight slowly on to it and as you do so, turn the rear right foot in so that it is at an angle of 45 degrees or so to the direction in which you are facing.

This sounds complicated but it isn't. Follow the instructions one at a time and you will find yourself once more in a Bow stance, left foot leading. Try this move often, experiencing the rotation as you turn your feet in. Once you can do it smoothly you will be able to make most of the transitions of the Tai Chi Forms quite easily. Do it starting from a right and left Rear stance.

5. You are once more on the railway lines. The image of the lines is merely a device to get you to keep your legs the width of your hips apart as you move. Once you can do this you can forget all about the image. Years of experience of teaching Tai Chi have shown me that this is one of the most difficult things for a beginner to remember. Stand in a right Bow stance. You are about to travel forwards in a different way from usual. Move into a Rear stance and turn your right toes out 45 degrees, placing the sole on the ground. Shift your weight on to this leg and bring the left foot close beside it, ball of the foot on the ground and heel raised, so that the ball of the foot is beside the right instep. Your body faces the same direction as your right leg. Then step forward into a left Bow stance, so that your body faces once more in the first, starting direction. Shift back into a Rear stance, turn the left foot out 45 degrees, put the sole down, bring up the right foot beside the left instep as before and step into a right Bow stance. The order is:

> Right Bow stance
> Right Rear stance
> Raise the right toes and turn out 45 degrees and put
>   sole on ground
> Shift weight on to right foot and bring left foot beside it
> Step into a left Bow stance, heel down first and 'rolling'
>   out the foot
> Repeat on the left side.

This mode of travel is the most common in Tai Chi. There are variations but once you can be familiar with this stance series and stepping action you will be able to follow the Forms with more confidence.

The next two exercises are to help you to slow down, inside yourself. One is an exercise I produced myself and the other comes from the training of Kyudo students. Kyudo is the Japanese form of ritualized archery. If you study them carefully you will acquire slowness and patience; very necessary in Tai Chi.

6. Stand with feet apart and parallel to one another. Take a full step forward with the right foot. Shift your weight on to it slowly. Bring up the left foot beside the right, parallel to it and 2 or 3 inches (5 to 8 centimeters) away to the side. It stops so that the tip of the left toes is opposite the middle of the right instep; no further. Most weight remains on the right foot. Pause for a second then *slide* the left foot so that the toes are in line with the right toes. Weight remains on the right foot. Slide the left foot a full foot's length ahead of the right foot and shift the weight on to it. Bring the right toes half way along to stop opposite the middle of the left instep. Pause a second. Slide the right foot so that the toes are in line with the left toes. Pause. Slide the right foot a full foot's length ahead of the left foot. Pause. Begin again.

> Full pace right – left toes half way along instep – left toes in line with right toes – left foot a full foot's length ahead – repeat on left side. Pause one second at least between each movement of the foot. The opening full pace with the right foot is not repeated.

When you move your foot, do so slowly and attentively, keeping your body relaxed. It is likely you will feel impatient with the exercise. Ignore this and continue for at least five minutes until you feel reconciled with the speed and action of the movement.

7. Stand with your feet apart and parallel to one another. Take a full step forward along the railway lines with the left foot, putting only the heel down. At this point *all* your weight is on the right foot. The left heel supports only the weight of the leg itself. Your left shin and ankle muscles are contracted to raise your toes; not a strong contraction, just enough to keep the foot in position. Slowly and with a firm intention relax your shin and ankle muscles to lower the sole of the left foot to the ground. The entire weight is still on the right leg. Most students, when they begin to learn this exercise, tend to shift the weight forward on to

the left foot as the sole of the foot is lowered. *Do not do this*. Only when the sole is fully lowered do you slowly shift weight on to the left foot. Feel the muscles of leg and foot begin to contract to support the weight and find balance. Relax the right leg as the left takes the weight and raise the right heel so that only the ball of the right foot rests on the ground. Repeat the exercise with the right foot in front.

A key point from an anatomical point of view in this exercise is that when you lower your front sole on to the ground you bend your rear supporting knee a little. If you do not do this you will have to stretch your front leg and this will upset things. Another point worth emphasizing is that when you lower the sole on to the ground you relax the shin muscle and ankle as much as you possibly can.

This exercise has been tried and tested. It is very beneficial. After five to ten minutes of its correct execution the legs begin to feel warm and relaxed as the additional blood and nerve circulation, the chi circulation if you will, builds up. This can extend to the upper legs and lower half of the torso as well. It is an excellent adjunct to Tai Chi training.

You should now, after the last two chapters, be able to devise variations on the different exercises presented. This will be helped if the exercises have done something to stimulate your interest in how your body works and to show you that moving more slowly than usual can produce a different kind of perception. With application you may come to accept this different perception and the benefits which it can bring.

7. Push Hands (Tui Shou)

Push Hands training is less well known in the West than the solo form of Tai Chi. It is a method of testing one's Tai Chi skill and understanding of principles.

During the last twenty-five years or so the form in which Push Hands training is done has widened, to encompass changes which were at one time unexpected. The form of Push Hands described in this chapter is the one which is generally recognized by students who stick to traditional methods. The arguments for and against change are long and involved and they can be found in martial arts magazine articles of the period concerned.

Push Hands is training undertaken with a partner. Using mainly the palms of the hands, contact is made between you and your partner, touching the wrists, forearms, elbows, upper arms, shoulders and trunk, in a definite way. Just as you have seen Forms demonstrated in the Set, so there are Forms of Push Hands. These Forms utilize the movements of the solo Forms and demonstrate how they *might* be used in defending yourself, and at a more sensitive level to demonstrate the interplay of Yin and Yang, tension and relaxation, vis-à-vis pressure placed on you by your partner.

Initially you have to feel your way, getting used to keeping your balance when your partner pushes against your raised forearm, and giving in to the push to neutralize his or her force. With training you learn to be able to cause your partner to lose balance by pushing as well as yielding. Fundamentally, yielding depends on your not allowing your partner any leverage or resistance. If a towel is hanging from a line and you push it, it offers little resistance. You study how to become like this towel, but in an alive way, not a dead way.

When you push you search for a point of resistance or lever-age on your partner's arms or body. Obviously it is far more difficult to yield with the body than with the arm, so students try to move in such a way that a partner cannot easily make contact with the body. But before such freestyle evasion enters the training programme there are various Forms which ensure a disciplined and safe approach. This is one of the values of Forms in martial arts training. Everyone knows what is going on and accidents are reduced.

Terms

Peng or Ward Off – is a movement from the Set. The forearm is raised across the front of the chest (Figure 89). Initially it is a defensive position. In quality it is like elastic water; it yields to a push but 'adheres' to it. When the push has been absorbed then Peng can as it were rebound and push away.

Li or Roll Back – also from the Set. The upper arm is horizontal and the lower arm raised 45 degrees ahead of the body (Figure 90). It is a deflecting or parrying movement, with the added purpose of drawing a partner in closer. In quality it is like guiding something to one side as one might divert the path of a small boat floating in the water.

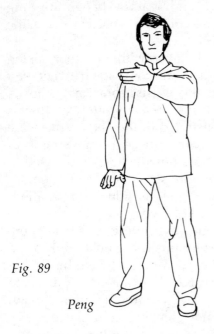

Fig. 89

Peng

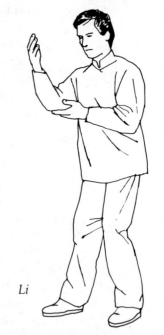

Fig. 90

Li

Ji or Press – a Form from the Set with both palms joined at the heels or wrists. Its action is to press forward against the partner's body, to send him or her toppling (Figure 91). In quality it is strong, persistent and searching.

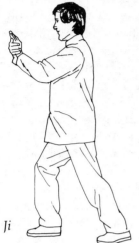

Ji

Fig. 91

An or Push – is found in the Set. Its action is to rest both palms on the partner's arms or body, and with the help of a push from the legs to uproot him or her, that is to disturb the balance to such an extent that the partner literally leaves the floor, sometimes (Figure 92). Its quality is to be irresistible, like a mounting wave.

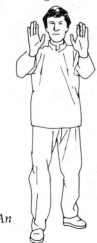

An

Fig. 92

Cai or Pull Down – comes in the Set and involves seizing hold of a partner's arms and, combined with a sinking of your body weight, to bring him or her forward and downward, off balance (Figure 93). Its quality is to be decisive and strong, tenacious and fast.

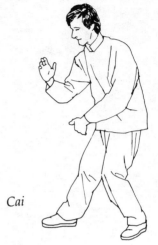

Cai

Fig. 93

Lie or Pull to Side – this move is found frequently in the Set as an intervening action between two Postures. It involves seizing a partner's arms at the wrist and elbow and diverting him or her to the side, at the same time pressing down to bring the partner off balance or even to the ground (Figure 94). Its quality is opportunist!

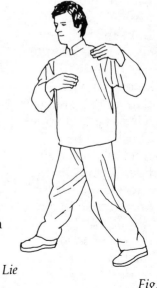

Lie

Fig. 94

Jou or Elbow – is a definite action from the Set. It is not used to its full extent in Push Hands as it means to strike in the solar plexus, for instance with the point of the elbow (Figure 95). In Push Hands the strike has to be restricted to a pushing action. In quality it is penetrating.

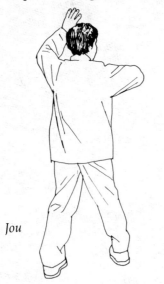

Jou

Fig. 95

Kao or Shoulder Stroke – a move from the Set. The shoulder is used to strike, body turned sideways on (Figure 96). Again it is not a technique which can be forcefully used in Push Hands as the effect can be harmful, so it should be restricted to a pushing action. Its quality is that of a battering ram.

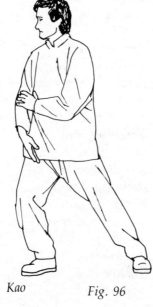

Kao   *Fig. 96*

The reason why the above techniques are favoured in Push Hands is that they exercise the energy in the optimum way, from a Tai Chi point of view. In Karate for instance certain kicks and punches are favoured because they have proved to be the most efficient. Ward Off and Roll Back help to circulate the Chi, out, in, out, in, utilizing waist, abdominal region, arms and hands so that energy can be absorbed and released according to Tai Chi principles. In this respect they are a form of Chi Kung. In Roll Back for instance you absorb; in Ward Off you release or expel. Chi comes in; Chi goes out; only to come in once more. The movement and the Chi move in a circle. When the whole body moves as one unit, the movement is a total or combined pattern which conforms to the movement of Chi. In Tai Chi classic writings it says that nothing can be added and nothing taken away, which means that everything involved in the movement is necessary, that nothing else is needed and that if any part of the movement were changed or left out then the result would not be the one which is required. Just as we could posit the notion that there is an optimum mode of breathing in any particular circumstance, but that it is rare that this mode is ever reached, so we can see that it will be rare for a Push Hands session ever to reach its ideal condition. Even so, the enjoyment or interest is in the striving, and studying.

Methods

1. Stand opposite your partner, both in right Bow Stance. Raise right wrists and rest the backs of the wrists against one another. Partner A turns his wrist

that his palm rests on the wrist of Partner B (Figure 97). Using his leg action as the initiator of movement, A pushes in a straight line against B's wrist. B yields by shifting weight backwards a little and turning to his left, diverting the push (Figure 98). A can go no further forward without losing balance. B turns his wrist so that his palm comes to rest on A's wrist. This is made possible by A turning his wrist so that his palm faces his body; that is, both wrists turn at the same time (Figure 99). B in turn pushes, and A yields. The cycle continues.

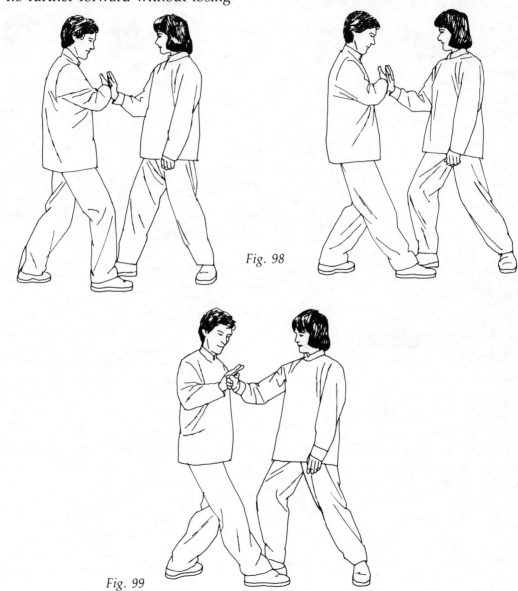

Fig. 97

Fig. 98

Fig. 99

2. Stand as in 1, but this time B presents his right arm in the Ward Off position, across his chest. A rests his right palm on B's wrist and his left on B's elbow, in Push position (Figure 100). A pushes forward in a straight line and B yields, turning to his left. When A can go no further without losing balance,

B turns his right palm to contact A's wrist, B having turned his palm towards his body to facilitate this, and brings his left palm to A's elbow (Figure 101). A also draws back his left palm in front of his left chest. Then B pushes, A yields and the cycle continues (Figure 102).

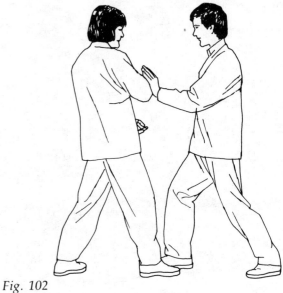

Fig. 102

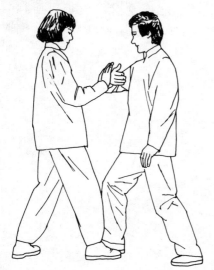

Fig. 100

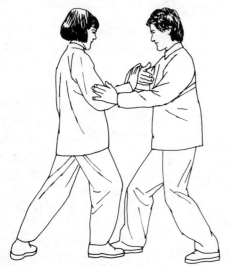

Fig. 101

These are the two basic methods of Push Hands. For a full presentation of Push Hands I refer readers to my book, *Tai Chi For Two*. When training, you try to be relaxed and aware of what is taking place. When the desire to 'win', push your partner over, and so forth, comes up, seek to avoid it and concentrate only on what is happening. Push Hands should be something you study; not a competition. Focus your mind on the interplay of Yin and Yang in your body and the body of your partner.

8. Tai Chi Today

I came across Tai Chi in 1968 at a demonstration given by Gerda Geddes, a well-known teacher. It was virtually unknown in England at that time. My first teacher was a pupil of T.T. Liang, perhaps the closest disciple of Cheng Man-ch'ing, and a master of Tai Chi in his own right. I learned Yang-style Long Form. This style and form is one of the most popular in the world today, though as the appetite for Tai Chi grows, other styles and forms are gaining ground. The Long Form is *long* . . . It needs plenty of patience and when I became a teacher of Tai Chi I usually taught the Cheng Short Form of Yang style to beginners. Then I learned Wu style of the Wu Chien Chuan line, from the daughter of a Hong Kong neurologist. My teacher did not recognize Yang style at all, presumably because she had never seen it. In later years I learned other forms and styles, realizing as I did so that Tai Chi Forms and Sets vary a great deal. For instance Yang style is slow, strong and flowing like a big river. Chen style is varied, changing in pace; now soft, now explosive.

Largely it seems from ignorance, a lot of misconceptions have been planted in people's minds about what is 'correct' Tai Chi. It is like deciding what is correct music. There is, in our society at least, no such thing. What there is to guide us are principles. Musical instruments must be in tune; the musicians must all be playing in the same key; they must all play at the same tempo, and so on. Similarly Tai Chi has its principles and it is they which determine what is Tai Chi. Along with these considerations is the question of quality. One violinist might play before the most discriminating of audiences and produce in them a sense of admiration, even awe. Another violinist on the same stage might drive every member of the same audience from the concert hall. But it is music in both instances. So, though standards vary, it is just as well to accept Tai Chi at whatever standard you find it. After all, it is something which people do for themselves, not for an audience.

Since 1968 Tai Chi has spread far and wide in the Western world. Some of my own pupils now teach Tai Chi. Their pupils may teach it also, and even their pupils may teach it. Each and every one of this group of people may have learned other forms of Tai Chi. Consider this on a worldwide scale and one can hardly begin to appreciate the diversity of large and small variations which have emerged.

When performing Tai Chi it is customary to wear loose-fitting clothing and flat-soled shoes such as gym shoes, Kung Fu shoes, soft casual shoes and so on. The ankle should be free to move and the sole of the shoe should be thin. As with most forms of exercise one tries to do it in a well-ventilated place or even outdoors weather permitting. There is a Chinese tradition of training under trees, since the tree is said to give out beneficial Chi which the student can absorb when breathing. It is not unusual these days to see people doing Tai Chi in parks and open spaces.

Diverse people produce diverse views and Tai Chi has not avoided this. Today we can find a number of views about the art. Sometimes one of these views is held to the exclusion of all others, and in other cases outlooks are so liberal that a person can hold all views simultaneously. Look at the following:

1. Tai Chi is a spiritual Taoist art and should only be approached in this light. It should never be used aggressively or competitively.
2. Tai Chi originated as a combative art and only later became a form of exercise and meditation in movement. It should stick to its combative roots.
3. Today people like to watch competitions, and to spread in popularity Tai Chi must have competitive forms and rules to attract the public.
4. Tai Chi should always be done in the same way out of respect for its founders and any departure from this way should be discouraged.

5. Tai Chi is subject to change and should develop when new ways of doing it are discovered.
6. Tai Chi is a Chinese art and Western people will never understand it.
7. Tai Chi is simply a part of the body-mind-spirit therapy movement and can be absorbed into any 'syllabus' of re-education that anyone cares to adopt.

These are perhaps the main views on Tai Chi currently held, though of course there will be others and combinations of the above. I now have no comment personally but only some food for possible thought to offer.

Tai Chi is a very personal thing, an intimate thing. It is to do with the circulation and use of your own energy, your Chi. A teacher can give only indications; the rest is up to you. In a society as intellectually and emotionally chaotic as ours, every system, every method gets sucked into this chaos. So if you are interested in Tai Chi you might consider trying to keep it outside all the pressures and mass compulsions which sweep through our society so that it is something which you do for yourself; something which is your own. This implies that you regard what other people do in the field of your art as merely food for thought and deliberation, not necessarily as an example to be slavishly followed. This of course includes what I say in this book.

To approach Tai Chi in this way requires a kind of discipline, an independence. You are then constantly learning and questioning what you do and why. Tai Chi can be kept separate from earning money, impressing members of the opposite sex, from conceit and egoism; in fact from everything else except its own principles. If you follow it in this way a time will come when you begin to see it as something strong and reliable in your life; something which contrasts with other things and throws light on them.

To do this requires training at the physical movements on a regular basis. It is not just an intellectual exercise. The physical training and the thinking should work together, in proportion. The softness of Tai Chi comes from rigour in training. If you are in 'normal' health but weak, physically lazy, dreamy, this is no good. You must go over the Forms repeatedly, seeing how they work, how they fit together, how each limb and part of the trunk move, how the weight changes, and so on. As you appreciate how the limbs work, you need relaxation, that is, an appreciation of the difference which comes to you when you are more relaxed. This should be treasured or at least respected, because it is one of the keys. If you do not find this you will be at a big disadvantage. I had a pupil who was recovering from a bad heart condition, and she found that by relaxing and then exerting certain muscles, combined with sending her Chi to certain parts of the body, her condition improved greatly.

There are many Tai Chi organizations throughout the world. In general they are based on commercial principles. This is understandable. Teachers cannot spend their time teaching for nothing. Organizations vary, from individual teachers running their own clubs in relative obscurity to ones which proclaim themselves as the British or International or All American or Pan European or some such grandiose title. The truth is that there is no organization for Tai Chi even remotely comparable with say the Amateur Boxing Association or the Amateur Athletic Association or the Rugby or Soccer leagues, the British Judo Association, and so on. All Tai Chi organizations are relatively small, and their titles in this sense are often a misrepresentation of their numerical size and unity. If you heard of say the Russian Tai Chi Association you would understandably believe it to be the representative body for the vast majority of Tai Chi practitioners in Russia. In Great Britain, where you might believe that an organization with a similar title represented the vast majority of British practitioners, you would be wrong. There are more students of Tai Chi in Britain who belong to no organization at all than there are students who do. The reason for this is that rules, organizing, form-filling and all the semi-hysteria that surrounds a great deal of sport is alien to Tai Chi. This is how things have turned out, and it is no reflection on the quality of teaching in organizations but merely an indication, in my view, of the very personal nature of Tai Chi.

In the last few years a tough form of Push Hands has gained in popularity, attracting people who like a bit of a 'fight'. The contests attract audiences and are often exciting. They resemble a watered down version of Japanese Sumo wrestling, and I suppose are roughly in line with the combative strand of Tai Chi which has existed for a long time. The contests require skill and determination. This said, there is a question mark hanging over them in the minds of the majority of Tai Chi students at this time (1993), because the majority do Tai Chi for relaxation and health, and the last thing on their minds at such times is being in an arena surrounded by hundreds of yelling people. Another question mark concerns combat itself. In internal arts it is possible to build up energy, Chi, to quite a degree. When this is combined with relaxation and good physical coordination the resulting applied force can be considerable. This force is less of a push or shove and more of an explosion or battering ram. It is not practical to use such techniques in a sporting context because people would be seriously hurt. This means that one of the more formidable uses of Tai Chi is excluded from competition. Some followers of traditional Eastern martial arts do not take part in competitions at all, as they consider that a martial art can never be a sport. Such attitudes are part and parcel of the endless discussions which occupy some of the time of martial arts enthusiasts.

How much time should you spend on training? Another question with no satisfactory answer. You get from Tai Chi, like everything else, what you put into it. An old Chinese friend of mine said he did Tai Chi twenty minutes before he went to bed because it helped him to relax, forget his daily routine, and sleep better. Other people do it early in the morning to start the day on a tranquil note. At one time in my life I did Tai Chi a great deal; hours every day, even in the dark in my garden. When you are learning the first parts of a Form or Set, as a beginner, you need daily practice, morning and evening I would say, to establish a new way of moving and to establish the physical memory of each movement. If you do not do this you will go to your weekly class or classes and every time have to relearn what you did in the previous session, wasting time and money and falling behind the more able members of the class. Once you get into the routine of your set you will probably find learning easier, because you will become accustomed to moving in the Tai Chi way both in terms of tempo and shifting of body weight. In this respect I recommend Tai Chi walking (see p. 83) as one of the first things that you do before commencing a Set or Form session.

Something worth mentioning is the cultivation of watching carefully when you are shown a Tai Chi movement by your teacher. Watch in several different ways. Look at the details: how the right arm moves, how the head turns, how the left foot steps and so on. Then disengage from watching one part and try to get a complete impression of the whole body and copy it, forgetting the details. You need both approaches. When looking at details you are trying for precision. When getting an overall impression you are trying for feeling or to be more precise a feeling-sensation of *how* the whole movement is being carried out.

Tai Chi is a rewarding study and an enjoyable one. If you have an affinity for it your life will be enriched.

Further Reading

Bow Sim Mark, *Combined Tai Chi*, Massachusetts, 1985.

Chuang Tzu, *Happy Journey or Excursion* (*see* Fung Yu-Lan).

Chung-Yan, *Creativity and Taoism*, Wildwood House, 1975.

Crompton, Paul, *The Elements of Tai Chi*, Element Books, 1990.

– *Animal Forms of Chi Kung*, PHC Ltd., 1993.

– *Tai Chi For Two*, Shambala, 1990.

– *Tai Chi Combat*, Shambala, 1991.

– *Tai Chi Workbook*, Shambala, 1987.

– *Chinese Soft Exercise*, PHC Ltd., 1986.

I-Ching, trans. Richard Wilhelm, Routledge, 1965.

Katchmer, George A., *The Tao of Bioenergetics*, YMAA, 1993.

Lao Tze, *Tao Te Ching*, Unwin, 1976.

Ouspensky, P.D., *In Search of the Miraculous*, Routledge, 1951.

Sun Tze, *The Art of War*, Cambridge University Press.

The Yellow Emperor's Book of Internal Medicine, California University Press, 1972.

Yu-Lan, Fung, *A Short History of Chinese Philosophy*, Macmillan, 1948.

Tai Chi & Internal Martial Arts Journal, Quarterly.

Useful Addresses

Tai Chi Union for Great Britain, 102 Felsham Road, London
SW15 1DQ

British Tai Chi Chuan & Shaolin Kung Fu Association, 28
Linden Farm Drive, Countesthorpe, Leicester LE8 3SX

General Index

acceleration 23
acupuncture 14
ankle 24
awareness 31

Bodhidharma xiv, 10
Bow Sim Mark xiii
Bow Stance 81–2

Ch'an Buddhism 10
Chang San Feng ix
chi 13
   types of 17
Chi Kung xiii–xv, 13
Combined Form xii
contending 2, 3, 6
Chuang Tzu 5

endorphins 14, 19
exercises 31

feet 79
Five Elements 8
Following Step 56
Forms 16, 23, 33, 42,
   91
   48 Forms 42
   definitions of 42

gravity 21, 25, 29–30

I-Ching 9

Lao Tzu 4, 5
Li Tian-ji xii–xiii

natural 5

physics 21, 27
   laws of 21
posture 42
principles 27
Push Hands 2, 6, 85–6

Rear Stance 81–2
Roll Back 22
root 4

Set 42
stance 22
styles xi
Sun Lu-tang xi
Sweep Lotus 23

Tai Chi, views on 92
tan tien 17
Tao Te Ching 2–3
Taoism 2
Taoist 18
Te 4–5
translations 42
Turned In Stance 81–2

Wang Tsung-yueh x
Ward Off 22
Wu-wei 3
Wushu xii

Yang 39
Yang family xi, xii, 42
Yin-Yang 2, 7, 9, 10, 28

Index of Forms

As If Closing A Door 68

Bend The Bow To Shoot
  The Tiger 77
Brush Knee and Punch
  Down 57
Brush Left and Right Knees
  67
Brush Left Knee and Twist
  47

Closing 79
Crossing Hands 78

Diagonal Leaning 53

Fair Lady Works with
  Shuttles 70
Fan Penetrates Back 66

High Pat On Horse 64

Kick With Left Heel 65
Kick With Right and Left
  Feet 66
Kick With Right Heel 64

Needle At Sea Bottom 66

Part Wild Horse Mane 63
Pat Foot To Tame Tiger 58
Play Guitar (left) 49
Play Guitar (right) 56
Preparation and Beginning
  45
Press Down Palms With
  Empty Step 71
Punch Under Elbow 54
Punch With Concealed Fist
  65
Push Forearm With Horse
  Stance 72

Single Whip (left) 48
Single Whip (right) 62
Single Whip Squatting
  Down 74
Stand On One Leg Holding
  Out Palm 72
Stand On One Leg To Ride
  The Tiger 75
Step Back and Whirl Arms
  65
Step Up and Cross Fists 75
Step Up and Punch 68
Step Back with Cross-over
  Palm 71
Strike, Parry and Punch
  (left) 51
Strike, Parry and Punch
  (right) 78
Strike With Both Fists 65
Stroke and Push 50

Sweep Lotus With Leg 76
Swinging Palms and
    Crouching Step 74

Threading Palm and Crouch
    Down 60
Turn and Push 55
Turn Left and Strike 60
Turn Body With Large
    Strokes 72
Turn Right and Strike 69

Ward Off, Roll Back (left)
    52
Ward Off, Roll Back (right)
    78
Ward Off Standing On One
    Leg 61
Wave Hands Like Clouds
    62, 69
White Crane Spreads Wings
    46
White Snake Puts Out
    Tongue 57